Disaster Management For Kids

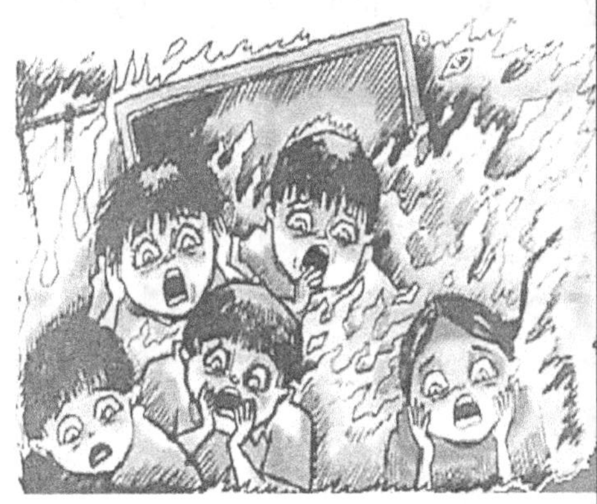

Christopher Fernandes
&
Dr. Fr. Francis Swamy S.J.

- 23rd December 1995, nearly 425 people, many school children perished in the flames during a school prize day celebration in Dabwali, Haryana.

- Kumbakonam fire tragedy in Tamil Nadu killed 93 school children, all below 11 years.

- On 26th January 2001, the Gujarat earthquake in Bhuj, many innocent school children died.

- 26th July 2005, the Mumbai flood, swept and killed many innocent school children.

- …Let us learn from earlier tragedies & make our society more resilient from disasters.

Published by:

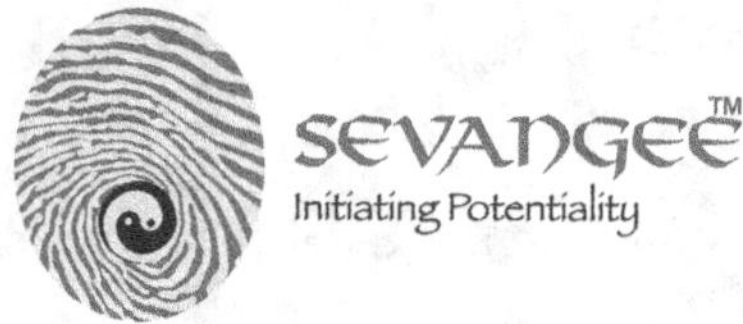

Main Office:

Sevangee Publications,
73, Sher-e-Punjab,
Andheri (East),
Mumbai 400 093
India
Contact: (+91) 8082555543

Printed in India.

Second Edition
ISBN No: 978-81-934689-1-3

Dedication

This book is dedicated to the countless heroes,
who have lost their lives in saving not only their loved ones,
but also the lives of others whom they did not know.
Life is precious, and
it is worth more than any other material things
this life or world can give us.

Acknowledgement

As molecules of atoms and ions form a compound, compounds form into dense matter, so also this book has gone through various phases and many great individuals and institutions have contributed their might, knowledge, time, energy, etc. A very big thanks to one and all.

Our sincere thanks to the Principal, Staff and Management of Apeejay High School, Nerul, Navi Mumbai, for helping, guiding and allowing us to browse through their library, and various other manuscripts of disaster management. Our sincere thanks to the Directorate General and the Commandant of Civil Defence for guiding us and sharing some of the techniques of evacuations. Our heartfelt gratitude to the Superintendent and the Staff of St. John's Ambulance, for sharing and giving us the details on first aid.

Our sincere thanks to the Staff and Management of Holy Family High School, Andheri (E), for giving us their unstinted support in this project. Our sincere thanks to Mr. Sanjay Jadhav, the Drawing Master of Holy Family High School, Andheri (E), for sketching out the excellent pictures here in. Our sincere thanks to Mrs. Collette D'souza the Ex. Vice Principal of Holy Family High School, Andheri (E).

Our sincere thanks to Mr. G. S. Sethi, who encouraged us and boosted us in doing this book and a very big thanks to his excellent staff of English Edition for helping us in doing the layout, proof reading, designing, etc. for without their help we would have been lost. Last but not the least we would like to thank our family members who have been a constant support, for without their help and encouragement we wouldn't have been able to accomplish this tack and make this book a reality.

Contents

‖ Introduction ‖

Creating a safe learning environment for children, is the most important task ahead. Recent events of children deaths due to natural disaster and manmade disasters like, building collapse, wall collapse, fire accidents, stampede, venturing in flooded zone, etc. brings the need to be continually vigilant, to ensure safety for students. The event that unfolded in the Kumbakonam fire tragedy in Tamil Nadu, which took 93 children to the jaws of death, the recent flood that captured the city of Mumbai, for more than twelve hours, the recent earthquake in Pakistan occupied Kashmir, are all eye openers, and it screams loud and clear, that it is high time we should have something called Disaster Management for Kids.

Disaster Management can be divided in three main components, these components are:

* The time before the disaster, i.e. the planning stage,
* During the disaster i.e. the evacuating stage and
* After the disaster i.e. the rehabilitation stage or giving first aid.

The likelihood of a natural or man made disaster related accidents are incalculable. Speculation may come without warning, in spite of several measures being drawn, many plans made, taking all precautionary measures, etc. Good plans are never finished, they can always be updated based on experience and changing vulnerabilities and assessment of current capabilities.

During the time of disaster, evacuation should be the prime goal of any disaster management techniques. Evacuation techniques are the heart and soul of disaster management. No matter what age or caste, creed or sex one belongs to, one has to know this skill of survival. Evacuating techniques comes in handy to evacuate the old, infirm, pregnant mother or lactating mother, the disabled, mentally or physically challenged, or the injured, depending upon the situation. Each life is precious, and it counts to make a city. We as human beings are joined in families, the families are joined in kinship groups, the kinship groups in clans, the clans in tribes, the tribes in nations, and that sense of hierarchy, of a pyramid in which layer upon layer is imposed. Hence life is precious, so we must take care.

After disaster has struck, thousands of people may be injured, but if you escape injury you can save the lives of others by giving first aid, before a qualified doctor arrives. Most of the injuries will be a peculiar type of nature like, people getting cut from flying glass, some may receive burns injury, some cases of fractured bones, many cases of bleeding or haemorrhage, some may have wounds and multiple injuries, some may have suffocation or unconsciousness. But remember: SHOCK WILL BE PRESENT IN ALMOST EVERY CASE. The idea of first aid is:

❀   to preserve life.

❀   to prevent the casualty's condition worsening.

❀   to promote recovery and save a life.

This book is primarily, targeted to promote a culture of disaster safety among the youth. It helps to inform, persuade, and integrate the issues of safety in disastrous situations. The goal of the book is to promote sensitivity, take proper safety measures and motivate key stakeholders through direct participation in activities that would foster towards forming a disaster resilient community. By educating children and building safety into their lives, we are ensuring a generation of future disaster managers, and building of a disaster resilient society. Remember, the time we spend on prevention today, may be the life we save tomorrow.

Chapter : 1

Understanding Disaster Management

Earth is a constant change, a battleground of natural forces between the internal (below the earth layer) and external (above the earth layer) forces. It is the work of these forces that rocks are deformed and made, soils are formed and destroyed, water on land and other resources are made available to us. Since human being reside both on dry as well as marshy land, they also come under the impact of these natural forces. The danger posed by these natural forces is termed as hazard. When under the impact of these forces loss of life and property is caused, it is termed as disaster.

Possibility of preventing Disaster :

It is through the natural forces that rocks and other materials are recycled to keep the earth robust and healthy. Our main concern is to know how the forces are manifested that pose danger to life on earth. While human beings cannot stop these natural forces from happening, they can certainly take measures to protect life, not only their own but also of plants and other animals. If nature is destroying one part of the earth, it is renewing another part. But man is only a destructive agent and that too in a very short period. These destructive man-made disasters are generally associated with pollution, cutting of trees, soil erosion, fires, dam failures, drought, gas and other chemical leaks including bombing, terrorism and other civil strifes. These are the main causes, which lead to major disasters. Disaster response is described as one's reaction to a disaster; it may even persist long after a disaster has struck.

Impact of Disaster :

◉ Disaster causes destruction of natural resources, life and property. As a result normal functioning of society is disturbed.

◉ Disasters gobbles up the wealth and property of people and the state in a matter of seconds.

◉ Hopes and expectations just evaporate into the unknown.

◉ Sometimes the victims have no other ways and means to claim compensation.

◉ An important environment consequence of a disaster is the damage caused to an ecosystem by pollution of rivers, ground water, dust and heat in the atmosphere.

◉ Difficulty to establish faults as a result of negligence or injury caused intentionally or un intentionally.

Guiding factor for Disaster :

◉ **Areas prone to Disaster:**

According to the theory of Continental Drift, the Indian peninsular is a part of the Gondwana landmass, which keeps moving towards the Tibetan region. Because of this drift, the whole Indian plateau keeps on shifting. Hence the Himalayan region is prone to earthquakes and landslides; the plains below have witnessed frequent floods and drought, while the coastal belts of Orissa, Andhra Pradesh, Gujarat and Tamil Nadu are faced with devastating cyclones and consequent floods and drought.

❖ **Location of residence:**

Certain locations like coastal areas are more vulnerable to cyclone than the interior region. The stormy winds of a cyclone may cause great damage to improperly built brick houses or a hut built of bamboo or other such materials. Geologically unstable areas, which are prone to earthquake, are not recommended for human settlement. Similarly, a steep-slope is more prone to landslides.

❖ **Density of Population:**

Densely populated areas are more prone to disaster, since too many infrastructure like, the electric poles, telephone poles, cables lines, old buildings, or poorly built structures are most of the time, disaster prone. A sudden damage or collapse of one of the above thing will ignite a chain reaction. More confusion is created by a mob than the actual disaster itself.

❖ **Threshold population :**

It is a population, which is living at the bottom, who relies heavily on a stimulus, to increase their strength to withstand natural or man-made disaster. This threshold population is supported by a fixed base, they comprise of women, especially pregnant and lactating mothers, children and old people, the disabled and mentally unstable people, poor and underprivileged classes, and uncomfortably large families.

❖ **Poverty :**

Poor people are more vulnerable to disaster, it is because their disaster-response is impeded by lack of resources.

These are some of the guiding factors, which multiply disaster. Disasters come in many shapes and sizes. Most are related to the weather. Some are predictable to a certain extent, like a cyclone. Some are not, like an earthquake, which really surprise us. Although disasters themselves aren't fun, but learning about them is really enjoyable. There is not much one can do about disaster, but there are things one can do to protect one's homes and reduce the risk of getting damaged. Reducing the risk is called "mitigation." However some mitigation is very expensive and complicated, like moving to a new home or to a different piece of land that is higher or away from a river, etc.

Causes of Disaster :

- Ignorance (cause, effect and redressal measures).
- Lack of Communication.
- Residing in Disaster prone locations.
- Unsafe residing structures (especially low income group).
- Lackadaisical approach towards nature & disaster.
- Imbalance of natural law or natural forces.
- Deforestation is the root cause of landslides.

Disaster can strike quickly and without warning. It can force you to evacuate the neighborhood or confine you to your home. What would you do if basic services like water, gas, electricity or telephones were cut off? Local officials and relief workers will be on the scene after a disaster, but they cannot reach everyone right away. Therefore, the best way is to make oneself self-reliant, your family and your home safer, and be prepared before disaster strikes.

Benefits of Disaster Management :

* Builds team spirit.
* Reduces impact of disasters.
* Makes one self-reliant. Builds Courage and Confidence.
* Builds Sensitivity towards others.
* Builds Awareness.
* Ignorance of disaster is perished.
* Redressal measures or mitigation.

Every family should have a Disaster Supply Kit in their home. The kit will help the family during a disaster. In a hurricane or earthquake, for example, one might be without electricity and the water supply may be polluted. In a heavy winter storm or flood, one may not be able to leave the house for a few days. In such times, one will need to rely on oneself. The disaster supply kit will make it easier. Remember, your family will probably never need to use the disaster supply kit, but it's always better to be prepared. It is best if these items are kept in a plastic tub or kept together in a cabinet so they will be easy to find.

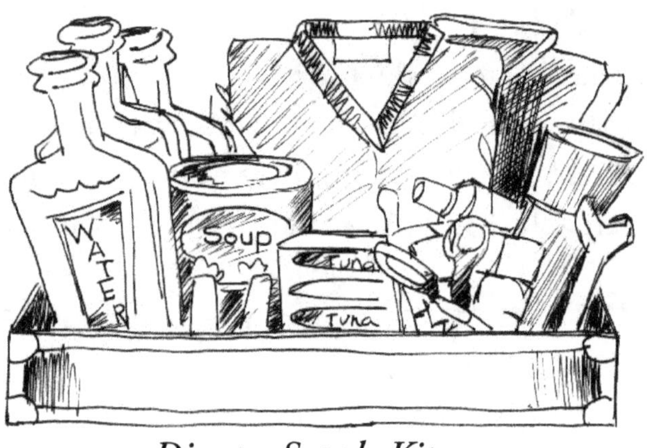

Disaster Supply Kit

Chapter : 2

‖ Earthquake ‖

Earthquakes are sudden shocks on the earth's surface. Earthquakes happen along 'fault lines' in the earth's crust. Earthquakes can be felt over large areas although they usually last less than one minute. It cannot be predicted, although scientists are working on it.

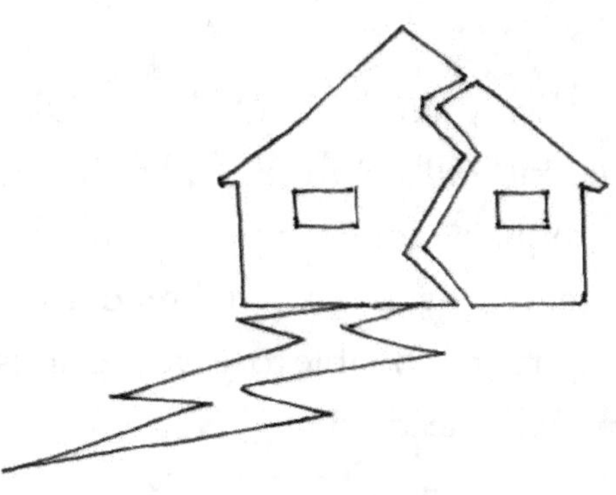

One may notice hanging plants swaying or objects wobbling on shelves. Sometimes you may hear a low rumbling noise or feel a sharp jolt. A survivor of the earthquake feels the sensation of riding a bicycle down a long flight of stairs-case.

Earthquakes themselves represent energetic condition of earth. Man however, has

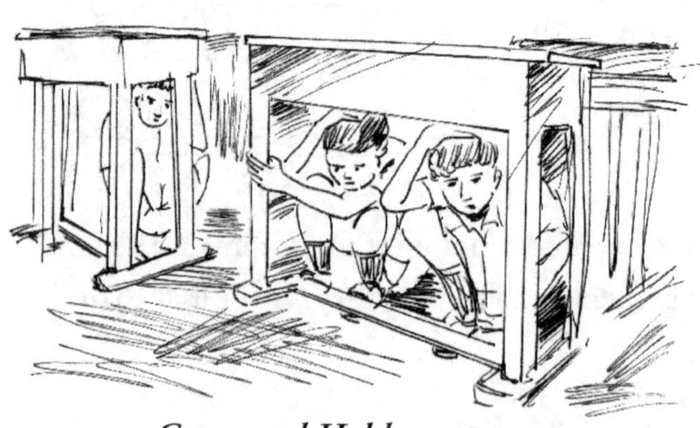

Cover and Hold on

not yet been able to invent any such instrument that can predict the sudden outburst of this energy. Only the intensity of the earthquake is measurable, one such measurement is called the Richter scale. Earthquakes below 4.0 on the Richter scale usually do not cause damage, and earthquakes below 2.0 usually can't be felt. Earthquakes over 5.0 on the Richter scale can cause damage. A magnitude of 6.0 on the Richter scale is considered strong and a magnitude 7.0 on the Richter scale is a major earthquake. Earthquakes are sometimes called temblors, quakes, shakers or seismic activity. The most important thing to remember during an earthquake is to DROP, COVER and HOLD ON. So remember to DROP to the floor and get under something for COVER and HOLD ON during the shaking.

Some Factors on Earthquakes :

❀ Earthquakes can happen anytime either day or night. There is no pattern.

❀ There is no connection between earthquakes and weather. Remember, earthquakes happen deep in the earth, far away from the weather.

❀ It seems like there are more earthquakes in recent times, but the truth is there are more reporting stations, and the media is more alert, than those previous years.

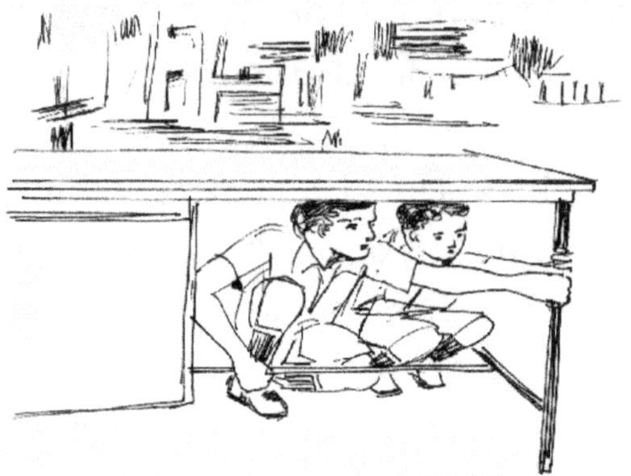

Drop, Cover and Hold

❀ One can protect one selves by securing a place where one stays, or the home where one lives. But remember earthquakes can't be prevented or predicted.

Things to do :

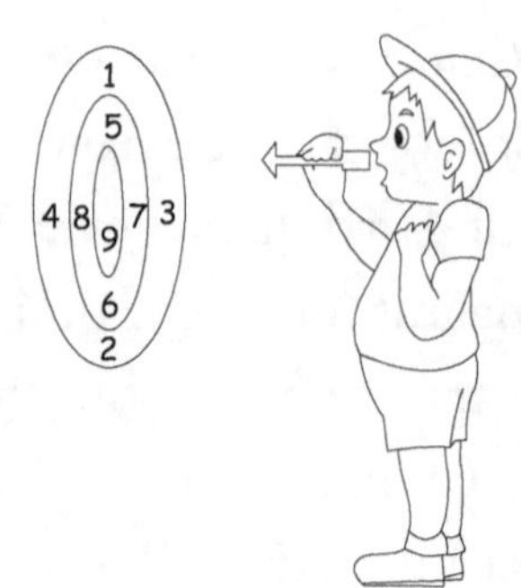

* If you are indoors during an earthquake, keep calm and take cover under a heavy table or desk. Stay away from glass windows or anything that could fall, like a book, case, cupboard, etc.

* If outdoors, move away from buildings, streetlights and utility wires.

* If caught in a crowded public place, do NOT rush for the doors. Everyone will be doing that. Instead, take cover under something heavy and stay away from things that could fall. Stay calm. Do not get in an elevator during an earthquake.

* After an earthquake, be prepared for after shocks. After shocks are follow-up earthquakes that are usually smaller than the first one. They are dangerous, because they cause things that are weakened in the previous quake, to crumble down.

* Bolt or strap cupboards and bookcases to the walls and keep heavy objects on the lower shelves, since after shock earthquake, things may tend to fall on people.

* If at home and one smells gas or hear a hissing or blowing sound, open a window and get out of the building right away. It may mean that a gas line in the house has been broken. Inform your parent or elders.

* Strap the water heater to a nearby wall. This will keep the water heater from falling on someone or starting a fire from a broken electric line.

☙   Make sure one is wearing shoes after an earthquake. There may be broken glasses scattered on the ground.

☙   If one is scared, share your fears with an adult. Earthquakes can be scary, but remember, they only last a few seconds.

Chapter : 3

‖ **Floods** ‖

Floods happen during heavy rains, when rivers overflow, there is an increase of water pressure in the reservoirs, strong winds, cyclones, tsunami, melting of glaciers, and ocean waves lashing on the shore, are all responsible for floods. When snowmelts too rapidly or when dams break, 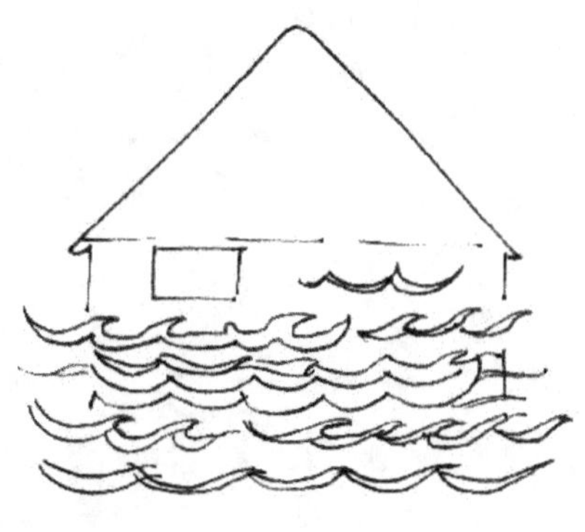 there is a tendency for flooding. It may be only a few inches of water or it may cover up, the roof. Floods are the most common natural hazards, that can occur in any state or cities.

Important terms to be known :

❁   **Flood Watch or Flashflood Watch :**

Floods that happen very quickly are called flashflood. Stay tuned to the radio or television news for more information. If one hears a flashflood warning, talk to elders immediately. Don't spread rumours.

❁   **Flood Warning :**

One may be asked to leave the area or get to a high ground right away, since the area will be flooded very soon. If possible tell an elder about the flood warning. If one has to leave the area, remember to bring the Disaster Supply Kit and make arrangements for pets, if any.

Things to do :

☀ If one has time, move important things to the higher floors.

☀ Don't put valuable items and appliances in the basement, since they are more likely to be flooded.

☀ Stay away from flood water. It may be contaminated (contain dangerous substances).

☀ Do not walk through gushing water. It can pull you off your feet. If you must walk through water, then move to an area where the force of water is fairly less. Use a stick to test the ground in front of you.

☀ If possible tie a rope where the water is gushing at high speed, so that many weak members can cross that area by holding on to the rope.

☀ Stay away from power lines that are on the ground. You could be electrocuted.

☀ Electricity and water don't mix. See that each house has a circuit breaker or fuse box and the utility meters are installed above the flood level for the particular area. In case there is a flood, water won't damage your utilities.

☀ Always keep your battery-powered radio with you, so you know what is happening.

◉ If you are scared, share your fears with an adult. Floods can be scary, but remember, the water ALWAYS goes away.

◉ Buy flood insurance. To learn more about flood insurance, have your parent call the insurance agency.

Chapter : 4

‖ Cyclone ‖

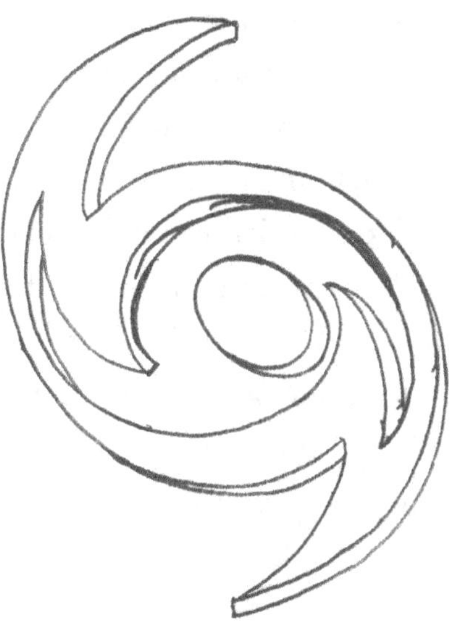

Cyclone is an atmospheric condition generally known as a storm. The low atmospheric pressure formed in the zone of disturbance area, separates the masses of cold and warm air, this warm air which is in the center, rises upward, and the cold air rushes in from all sides to take its place. The swirling winds at the center keep moving upwards at a velocity of 50 km or more an hour. This swirling motion is affected mostly by the earth's rotation in the tropical latitude areas. Tropical cyclones are called hurricanes. Hurricanes gather heat and energy through contact with warm ocean waters. Evaporation from the seawater increases their power. Hurricanes rotate in a counter-clockwise direction around the center, it has wind, which moves roughly at the speed of 74 miles per hour. When they come on land, the heavy rain, and strong winds can damage buildings, trees and cars. The heavy waves from the sea are referred as a storm surge. Storm surges are very dangerous and are a major reason why one MUST stay away from the ocean during a hurricane warning.

Why Can't We Stop Cyclones or Hurricanes?

One of the most commonly asked questions is why we don't try to stop cyclones or hurricanes from forming or disrupt them once they are formed. So far researchers have found it, impossible to do. The weather systems that make up hurricanes are too large to affect this. Most coastal areas in the world prone to cyclones, are the Caribbeans region, the coasts of Central and North America, India and China. Some of these countries have a network of stations to monitor the onset of cyclones. Satellite tracking the movement of cyclones can show their path accurately. Based on these tracking devices and meteorological recording instruments, it is likely to issue the onset or warnings, and also the severity of weather conditions like cold, heat, snow, etc. are predicted and announced on radio, television or through print media. In the United State of America, researchers have acquired airplanes to use for hurricane research. Improved computers and regular flights of 'Hurricane Hunter' planes help meteorologists (scientists who study weather) to learn more and more about hurricanes. Nowadays, the forecasts and project 'track' of hurricanes have become more accurate. In India there is a remote possibility of a Hurricane coming in, but it all depends upon the weather pattern. The recent depletion of ozone layers, have changed the weather pattern and it is becoming difficult to predict the weather.

Things to do :

* Don't let the roof be blown off by high winds. Have strong straps installed to keep the roof attached to the walls.
* Use storm shutters to protect windows and glass. Use them when

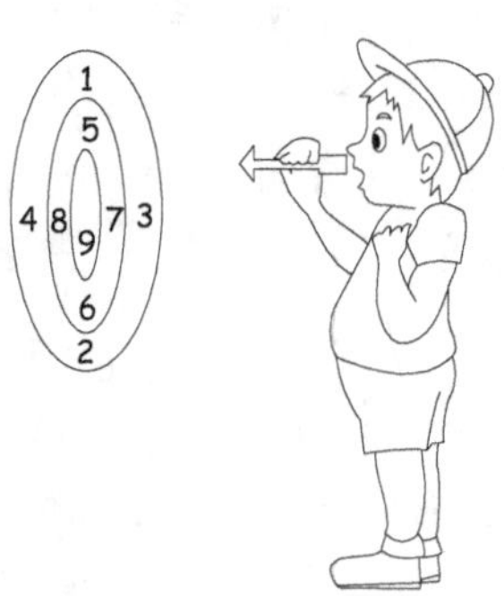

severe weather is forecast. The storm shutters protect against flying debris like tree trunks or other things carried by strong winds.

* Listen to a radio or television for weather updates, and stay in touch with neighbours and be prepared for evacuation orders.

* Plan a place to meet with family members in case if separated during a disaster. Choose a friend or relative from a different state or district, to call or to enquire, whether everything is OK.

* Get the disaster supply kit ready, store extra water, check if there is enough provisions of food and clothing.

* If possible try to remove the antennas from the roof, with the help of an adult.

* Shut off all utilities, like water, electricity and gas.

* Make sure there is fuel in the car so that you are ready to evacuate immediately, if you are told to do so.

* If you don't need to evacuate, be sure to STAY INDOORS during a cyclone. You could be hit by flying objects. Don't be fooled if there is a pause in the wind. It is the eye of the storm, and the winds will come again.

* Avoid using the phone keep it for emergency purpose.

* If you do evacuate, do NOT go back home, until local authorities say it is safe.

* Cyclones can be very scary. If possible try to talk to some adult about it.

Chapter : 5

▐▌ Thunderstorm or Lightning ▐▌

People who have been struck by lightning are safe to handle, they don't carry any electrical charge. Lightning cause burns, damage to the nervous system, broken bones, loss of hearing and maybe loss of eyesight.

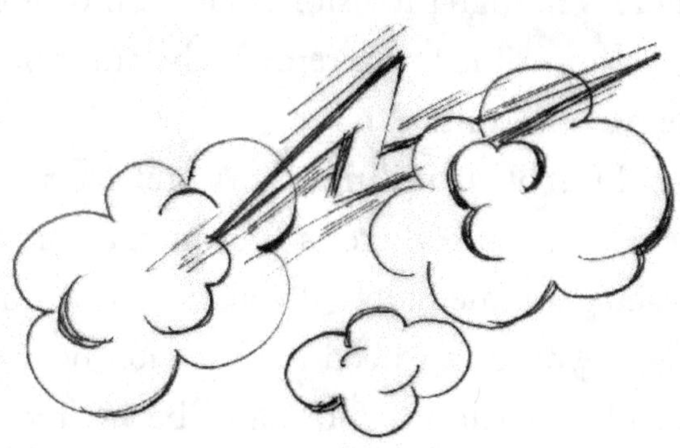

It is a very serious emergency. If you know how to give first aid and the person concerned has stopped breathing, then start giving mouth-to-mouth respiration. If their heart has stopped beating, and you know how to give Cardio Pulmonary Resuscitation, please do the needful at the earliest.

Thunder won't hurt, but lightning does. It is important to pay attention, when one hears thunder. Thunderstorms happen in every state and every thunderstorm has lightning. Lightning can strike people, buildings and it is very dangerous. Thunderstorms affect small areas when compared with hurricanes and winter storms. The typical thunderstorm is 15 miles in diameter and lasts for an average of 30 minutes. Nearly 1,800 thunderstorms are happening at any moment around the world.

Despite their small size, all thunderstorms are dangerous. Every thunderstorm produces lightning, which kills many people more people. Heavy rain from thunderstorms can lead to flash flooding. Strong winds, hail, and tornadoes are also dangers associated with some thunderstorms. Lightning is seen before thunder is heard, because light travels faster than sound.

Thunderstorm need three things :
* Moisture - to form clouds and rain.
* Unstable Air - relatively warm air that can rise rapidly.
* Lift - it lifts sea breezes and mountains helps in lifting the air to form thunderstorms.

Thunderstorms are most likely to occur in the spring and summer months, but they can occur all the year-round. Along the Gulf Coast and across the Southeastern and Western states, thunderstorms do occur during the afternoon. Thunder and lightning are accompanied with snowstorm, at high altitude region.

What Is Lightning?
The action of rising and descending air within a thunderstorm separates positive and negative charges. Water and ice particles also affect the distribution of electrical charge. Lightning results from the buildup and discharge of electrical energy between positively and negatively charged areas. Most lightning occurs within the cloud or the area between the cloud and the ground surface.

The average flash of lightning could turn on a 100-watt light bulb for more than 3 months. The air near a lightning strike is hotter than the surface of the sun. The rapid heating and cooling of air near the lightning channel causes a shock wave that results in thunder. Your chances of being struck by lightning are estimated to be 1 in 600,000 but following the safety rules one can reduce the chances of being struck by lightning. Most lightning deaths and injuries occur when people are caught outdoors, and it happen before or after rainfalls.

Facts on Lighting :

* Lightning has 'favourite' sites, it may hit continuously or many times at a particular area.

* Lightning often strikes when there is no heavy rain and it may occur as far as 10 miles away from any rainfall area.

* Rubber-soled shoes and rubber tires provide NO protection from lightning. However, the steel frame of a hard-topped vehicle provides increased protection if you are not touching metal. Although you may be injured if lightning strikes when you are in the car, but you are much safer inside a vehicle than outside.

* Lightning-struck victims do not carry any electrical charge and they should be attended immediately.

* What is referred, as 'heat lightning' is actually lightning from a thunderstorm too far away for thunder to be heard. However, the storm may be moving in your direction.

Things to do :

* When a storm is coming, look for darkening skies, flashes of light or increasing wind. Listen for the sound of thunder. If you can hear thunder, you are close enough to the storm to be struck by lightning. Go to safe shelter

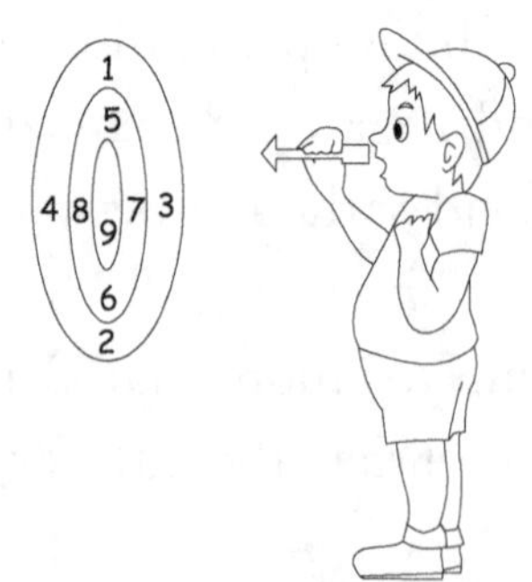

immediately. Find shelter in a building or car. Keep car windows closed and avoid convertibles.

* Telephone lines and metal pipes can conduct electricity. Unplug appliances, avoid using the telephone or any electrical appliances. (Leaving electrical lights on, however, does not increase the chances of your home being struck by lightning).

* Don't take a bath or shower.

* Turn off the air conditioner. Power surges from lightning can overload the compressor and damage the air conditioner.

* Draw blinds and shades over windows. If windows break due to objects being blown by the wind of a storm, then the shades will prevent glass from shattering into your house.

If you are caught outdoor during a thunderstorm, react immediately:

* If you are in the woods, take shelter under the short trees.

* If you are boating or swimming, get to land and find shelter right away.

* If you can go to a low-lying, open plain away from trees, poles or metal objects it is much safer. Make sure the place you pick is not subject to flooding.

* Become a very small target, squat low to the ground, place your hands on your knees with your head between them. Make yourself the smallest target possible.

* Do not lie flat on the ground, this will make you a larger target.

Chapter : 6

▎▎ Volcanoes ▎▎

A volcano is a mountain that opens downward to a pool of molten rock below the surface of the earth. When pressure builds up, eruptions occur. Gases and rock shoot up

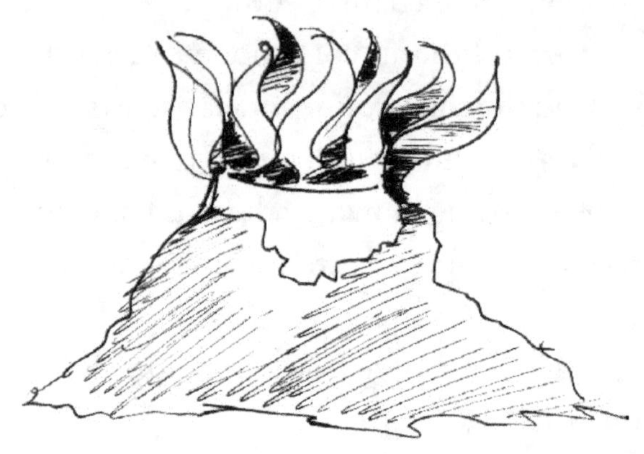

through the opening and spill over, filling the air with lava fragments. Eruptions can cause lateral blasts, where lava will flow with hot ash. Volcano eruptions have been known to knock down entire forests. An erupting volcano can trigger tsunamis, flashfloods, earthquakes, mudflows and rock falls. The danger area around a volcano covers about a 20-mile radius. Fresh volcanic ash, is made of pulverized rock, it can be harsh, acidic, gritty, glassy and smelly. The ash can cause damage to the lungs of older people, babies and people with respiratory problems.

Some Facts on Volcanoes :

❀ More than 80 percent of the earth's surface is volcanic in nature. The sea floor and mountains were formed by countless volcanic eruptions. Gaseous emissions from volcano formed the earth's atmosphere.

* May 18, 1980 eruption of Mount St. Helena in the Cascade Range of Washington State happened after more than 100 years of dormancy (a time when the volcano was 'asleep').

* There are more than 500 active volcanoes in the world. More than half of these volcanoes are part of the 'Ring of Fire' a region that encircles the Pacific Ocean.

* The rock debris carried by a lateral blast of Mount St. Helena travelled as fast as 250 miles per hour.

* Crater Lake in Oregon, USA, formed from a high volcano that lost its top after a series of tremendous explosions about 6,600 years ago.

Things to do :

* Do not visit the volcanic site. A sudden explosion could kill you. Officials posted there, may tell you the safest place to view.

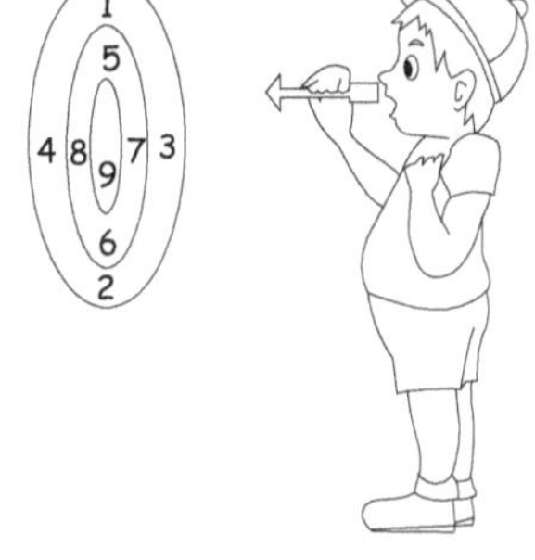

* If there is ash in the air, avoid being downwind from the volcano. A building offers good shelter from volcanic ash, but not from lava flow or rocks. If ash is falling, stay indoors   unless there is a danger of the roof collapsing. Close doors, windows and all ventilation in the house. Cover your nose and mouth to avoid breathing ash.

* Be aware of flying rocks and mudflows. Mudflows can move faster than you can walk or run.

* If you live near a volcanic region, you should have an evacuation plan. One should be very clear to which route one will

take if one has to evacuate and also have a back-up route.

   If one lives near a volcanic region, it is better to have a pair of goggles and a throwaway breathing mask for each member of the household.

❊   After an eruption, if you have ash on the roof, clear it away as soon as you can. The ash is heavy and could cause the roof to collapse.

‖ Tornadoes ‖

Tornadoes come from powerful thunderstorms and appear as rotating, funnel-shaped clouds with winds reaching up to 300 miles per hour. Tornadoes cause damage when they touch down on the ground, and the area they cover is approximately, one mile wide and 50 miles long. Severe weather can be very scary, but tornadoes are one of nature's most violent storms. Every country is at some risk from tornado damage, but countries like the United States of America and Canada have the highest risk, because of the Labrador currents. Tornadoes can form any time of the year, but the typical season runs from March to August.

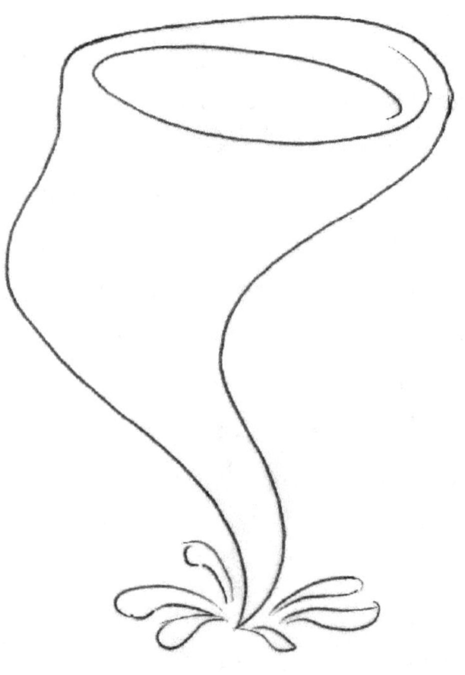

What should I do if a tornado is coming my way?

Tornadoes are hard to predict, one may get a few minutes warning. The most important thing to do is TAKE COVER when a tornado is nearby. It is also important to know the difference between a tornado watch and a tornado warning. A tornado watch is when tornadoes are possible in the area. No tornado has been spotted, but it could happen. A tornado warning is when a tornado has been seen, and one should take shelter immediately in a place without windows, such as bathroom or the basement.

Things to do :

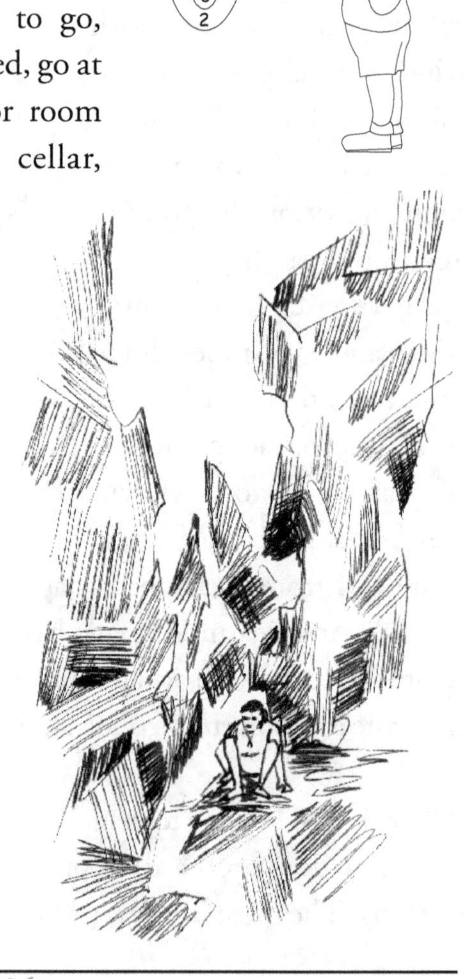

◉ Keep ears open, listen to weather forecast or weather updates.

◉ Be prepared as to where to go, when a tornado warning is issued, go at once to a windowless, interior room such as bathroom, storm cellar, basement or lowest level of the building.

◉ Make a list of items to bring inside in the event a tornado watch is issued. Don't forget the pets.

◉ Help parents and elders to trim diseased or damaged limbs from trees and shrubs and remove debris from the yard.

◉ Talk to your parents about having a plan for shelter and an out-of-state or district family contact in case one must relocate after a disaster.

Don't lose roof to high winds. See that your parents install strapping to keep the roof attached to the walls.

If you are at school during a tornado, listen and do what your teacher says.

If you are outside and cannot get inside, lie flat in a ditch or ravine. Lie face down and cover your head with your hands.

If you are in a car, take shelter in a nearby building.

After a tornado, watch for broken glass and power lines that are downed. If you see people who are injured, don't move them unless they are in a danger zone. Call for help right away.

Tornadoes can be very scary. If you are scared, be sure to talk to someone about it.

‖ Tsunami ‖

Tsunami (pronounced soo-nahm-ee) is a series of huge waves that happen after an undersea disturbance, such as an earthquake or volcanic 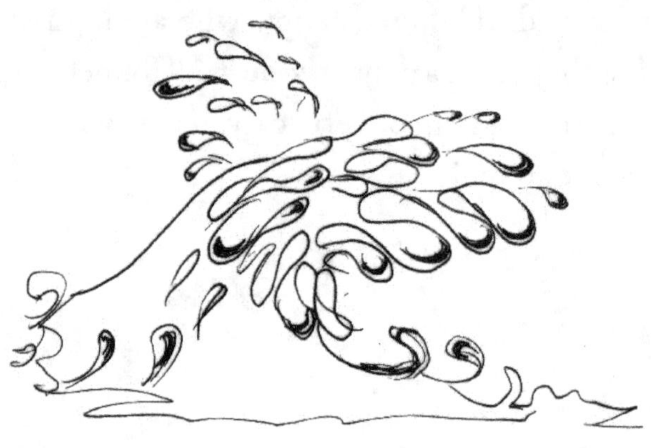 eruption. (Tsunami is from the Japanese word for harbour wave.) The waves travel in all directions from the area of disturbance, much like the ripples that happen after throwing a stone in water. The waves may travel in the open sea as fast as 450 miles per hour to more than 700 miles per hour. As the big waves approach shallow waters along the coast, they grow to a great height and smash into the shore. They can be as high as 100 feet. They can cause a lot of destruction on the shore. Sometimes they are mistakenly called 'tidal waves', but tsunamis have nothing to do with the tides. A tsunami is a series of waves, not a single wave, and the danger may not be over when you think it is. Hawaii is the state at greatest risk from tsunami. They experience about one a year, with a damaging tsunami happening about every seven years. A

Tsunami Warning Centers in Honolulu Hawaii and Palmer Alaska, monitor disturbances that might trigger a tsunami. When a tsunami is recorded, the center tracks it and issues a warning when needed.

Things to do:

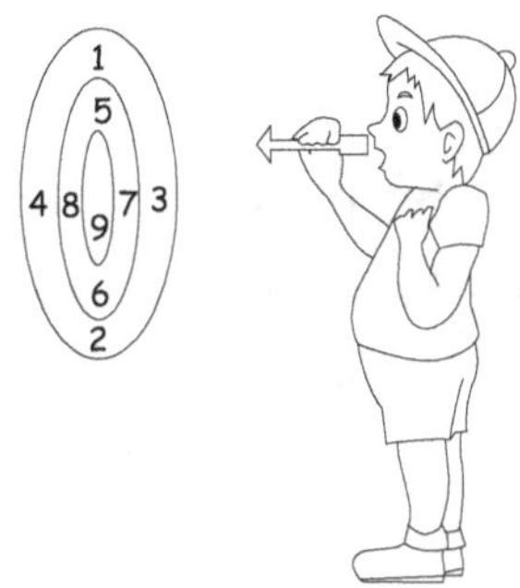

❀ Listen to your battery-powered radio if there is a tsunami warning. If you hear a tsunami warning, and they say to evacuate, do this immediately. Have an evacuation plan.

❀ A small tsunami at one beach can be a giant wave a few miles away. Do not let the small size of one wave make you forget how dangerous tsunamis are. The next wave could be bigger. Get away from the shoreline right away. When you see a tsunami it is too late to escape. Stay away until you hear the 'all clear' signal from the government officials.

Chapter : 9

▌▌ Winter storms ▌▌

In many northern areas of the Indian peninsula, winters bring heavy snowfall and very cold temperatures. Heavy snow can block roads and cause power lines to fail. The cold temperatures can be dangerous if one is not dressed properly.

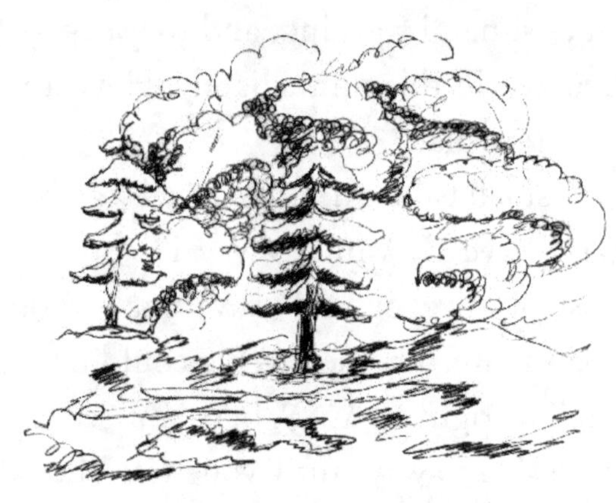

Some Important Terms :

Freezing rain :

Rain that freezes when it hits the ground, creates a coating of ice on roads and walkways.

Sleet :

Rain that turns to ice pellets before reaching the ground. Sleet also causes roads to freeze and become slippery.

Winter Storm Warning :

Cold, ice and snow are expected, on severe winter conditions.

Severe weather such as heavy snow or ice is possible in the next coming day or two.

Blizzard Warning :

Heavy snow and strong winds will produce blinding snow, near zero visibility, deep drifts and life-threatening wind chill.

Frost/Freeze Warning :

Below freezing temperatures are expected.

Things to do :

Be prepared for winter storms by having:

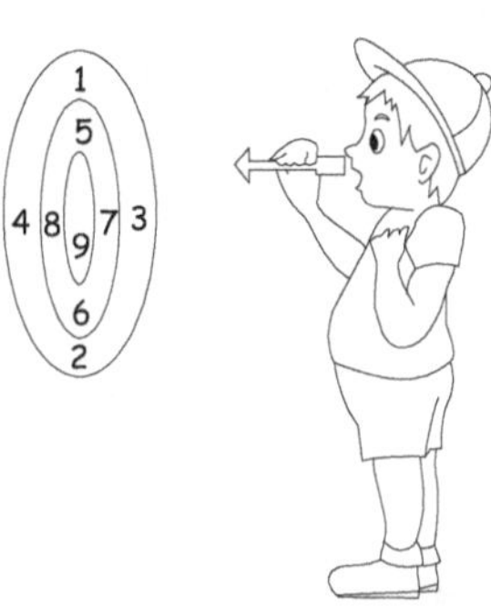

* a battery-powered radio with extra batteries,
* extra food that doesn't need cooking (like canned food),
* rock salt to melt ice and sand to improve traction,
* flashlights and battery-powered lamps (if the electricity goes off),
* wood for the fireplace (if you have one).
* If you go out in very cold weather, dress in several layers of clothing. Mittens are warmer than gloves, an one should wear a hat and cover the mouth with a scarf to protect the lungs from the cold air. Watch for frostbite.(Frostbite happens when the skin is exposed in very cold temperatures or one is not dressed warmly. One will experience a loss of sensation in that part, usually a finger or toe or the tip of the nose, and it may turn white or pale. Get immediate help).
* If you get trapped in your car during a blizzard, you should set

your lights on flashing and hang a piece of cloth or distress flag from the radio antennae or window. Then get back in and stay in the car. Do not go out on foot unless you can see a building nearby. Run the engine and heater about 10 minutes out of each hour. When the engine is running, open a window slightly. This will protect you from carbon monoxide poisoning. You may need to clear snow away from the car's exhaust pipe.

❀ You can use road maps, seat covers and floor mats for warmth. You can also huddle with the other passengers. Take turns sleeping so one person is always awake when rescuers come.

❀ If you are stranded in a remote area you may need to leave the car on foot after the blizzard passes.

Chapter: 10

‖ Fire and Wildfire ‖

Some common manmade disasters are fire, terrorism, chemical and industrial accidents, epidemics, nuclear accidents, war, etc.

Fire is a visible flame accompanied by heat, light, and smoke generally identifies fire. In reality fire is a chemical reaction

producing gas or vapour and accompanied by heat. The atoms or molecules in vapour are excited to high state of energy. This energy is released in the form of heat and light. It can be destructive if let loose while combining with oxygen in air, since there will be rapid reaction. For any reaction to spread it must be in contact with inflammable substances like wood, petrol, gas, coal, paper, plastics and even steel. The combustible materials also include many types of chemicals and minerals like for e.g. a match head, paints, varnish, etc.

If any of these three constituents of fires are removed, the fire will be extinguished. Fire spreads very rapidly, small fires causes big fires, therefore it is essential that small fires are extinguished immediately, and are not allowed to spread. There are many instances when fire can be accidentally ignited or lit by a burning cigarette butt coming in contact with any inflammable substance, or an electric spark may burn the wire and spread further. It is very important to prepare for both building fires and wild fires. Fires in buildings are very dangerous. Every year, fires kill more than 5,000 people in this country. Nowadays many new high-rise buildings have a smoke detectors or fire extinguishers. Look around for the smoke detector or fire extinguisher, check with your parents or any adult if the smoke detectors or the fire extinguishers are in working conditions. Have a fire plan of how to escape from the house if it is on fire. If you are caught in a fire REMEMBER, to stay low to the ground where the smoke is not so heavy, since air is heavier than gas. NEVER hide during a fire. Always get out, and once you are out, stay out. DO NOT go back for a toy. Tell an adult if there is a person left behind in the burning house.

Only You Can Prevent Wild Fires :

Wildfire is one of the most destructive natural forces on the planet. While sometimes lightning causes it, and other times it is caused by careless people, nine out of ten wildfires are due to human error. Wildfires are a danger to people who live in forests, prairies or wooded areas. These fires are sometimes started by lightning or by accident. They can move very fast and burn many acres. Remember, if there is a wildfire near you and your family and you are told to evacuate, go immediately, and remember to bring the pets with you. Wildfire experts say there are four reasons why wildfires happen more often:

a. The way forests were handled in the past, allowed fuel in the form of fallen leaves, branches and plant growth, to accumulate, this fuel fed the wildfire.

b. Increasingly hot, dry weather also gave reason for wild fire.

c. Changing weather patterns across the country.

d. Now a days more homes are built in the areas where wildfires occur.

Things to Remember :

Wild fires can be prevented, thus:

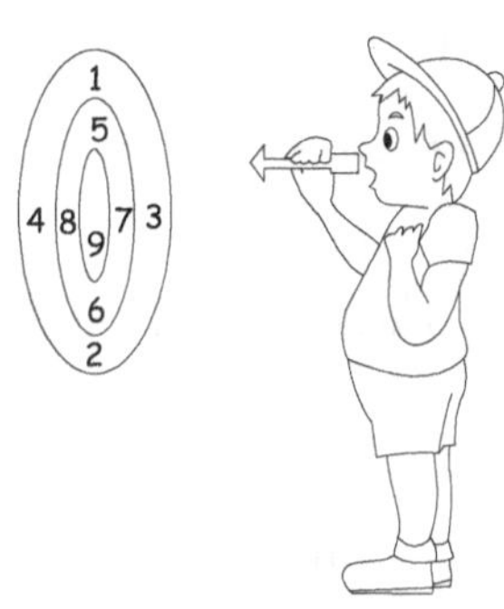

❖ By being careful with lighted cigarette butts, especially in the open or outdoors. They should be carefully extinguished and disposed of.

❖ See that cars and trucks are not parked near dry grass regions.

❖ Never burn trash in a haphazard manner.

❖ While camping inspect the campsite and ensure no fire is out of control.

❖ Never pull burning sticks out of a fire.

❖ Create a safety zone around the house that separates your home from plants and bushes that can burn easily. Clear dead bush and grass from your property. It will act as fuel for a fire.

❖ Keep branches around your home free of dead or dry wood or moss.

❖ Never burst any type of fireworks in a crowded place, always burst it in an open ground.

❖ Keep stoves, lanterns and heaters away from things that can catch fire.

- Always store containers with flammable liquids, in a safe place.
- Never use stoves, lanterns or heaters inside a tent.
- Evacuation is the first step and all routes to be decided on the spot.
- During evacuation dense smoke filled corridors must be avoided.
- Every one must have a basic knowledge of how to operate the fire extinguishers. It should be mandatory in all risk prone areas.
- Shut off gas cylinder immediately after use or while leaving the house or the laboratory. Similarly, matchboxes must be kept away from burning flames. Electrical appliances of all kinds like heater, cooker, iron or press, washing machine, radio, television, etc., must never be left unattended.

Chapter: 11

▌ Chemical Leakages ▐

The patterns of industrial hazards reveal that they can be sudden, slow or may not respond to any definite onset pattern. Though industrial establishments have their own 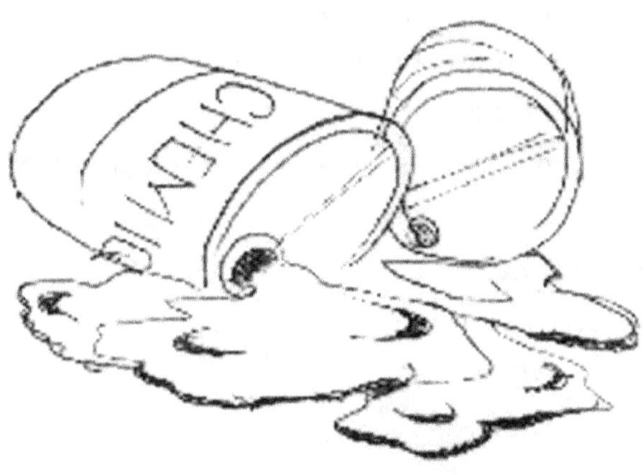monitoring and warning systems of gas/chemical leaks or accidents, they do not have basic mechanism to build up defences against disasters at short notice. They also often tend to ignore such warnings. In case of chemical leaks and industrial hazards, the most affected are pregnant women and lactating mothers (they have negative biological response to certain chemicals), accompanied with old people and young children too. The major portion of environment, land, water, and air are affected by chemicals leaks, since hazardous substances released in air and water, travel long distances and affect many people who come in contact with such water or air. It also affects the biological world in many different ways. Certain chemicals may produce long-term reactions and affect through inheritance, or they are pretty potent to cause debilitating disabilities like blindness, deafness, paralysis and nervous disorders.

Hazard of Chemical leakages:

Inhalation of such gases may cause cancer, stomach problems, heart and lung problems and even death. Eye exposure may damage eyesight temporarily or permanently. Skin exposure may cause skin cancer, irritation or other damage, malfunction of immune system and its damage may increase future risks. Even to some extent buildings are damaged permanently, like disfigurement of marbles, wooden furniture and fixtures.

Things to do :

* Heed warnings seriously and move to the predetermined zone as demanded by the authority.
* Remember to lie low in such incidents, since air is heavier than gas.
* While evacuating try to tie a wet cloth over the mouth and nostril region, since the dampness may try to filter some of the toxic air.

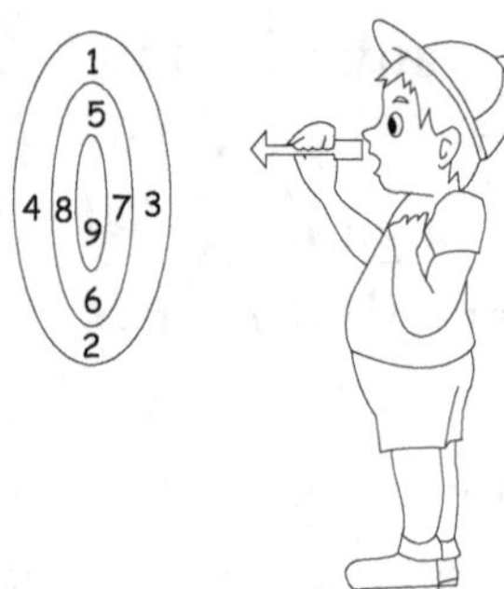

Chapter : 12

▍ Air raid or Bombing ▍

During war every aspect of life of a community is upset, it is therefore necessary for every man, woman and child to voluntarily join hands in a collective effort to protect themselves and their neighbours and keep their community life going as best as they can. Enemy air raids create complex and difficult problems, some of them are:

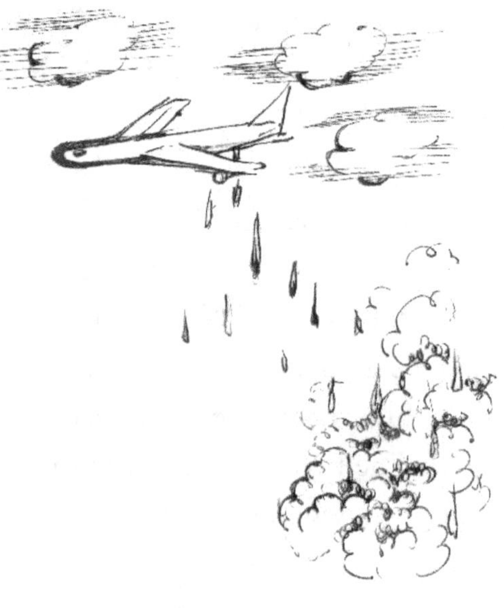

- Many people and animals either dead or injured.
- Buildings may be damaged, and many people could be buried under the debris.
- Essential services may be damaged.
- Large scale fires.
- People are rendered homeless and without food and clothing, family members are separated.
- Panic and rumours, aimless evacuation.

❀   Law and order problems.

❀   Unsanitary conditions and epidemics.

Although we are living in the Nuclear Age, yet the Conventional weapons, like the High Explosive and Incendiary Bombs, still play a major role. Even in the case of Nuclear weapon, the type and extent of damage, beyond the area of total destruction is similar to the destruction by the conventional weapons. Hence learning to prepare with the problems of conventional weapons can help to minimize the effect of attack, of an air raid or bomb attacks.

High Explosive Bomb :

High Explosive Bomb is a strong steel casing containing high explosive substance (TNT is generally used), fitted with a device for carriage by an aircraft, and the device of producing the spark to detonate high explosive substances and explode the bomb when required. The high explosive bomb contains a fuse, which can be made to work when the bomb is about to hit the target or when it hits the target and even after a short or long delay after hitting the target. The long delay may be for a few days, and the bomb may weigh from 10 kilograms to 10,000 kilograms. The bombs being dropped from high altitudes produce heavy loads on the structure where they hit. Depending on the construction of the bomb, like pointed nose, stronger casing, the bomb could damage many structures before it explodes. The important factor of the explosion is the blast. When the high explosive substance in the casing of the bomb starts burning, it turns from solid to explosive gas form. The casing expands and then breaks when the pressure of the gas inside is in the vicinity of about 500 tons per sq.inch. This compressed gas when liberated, causes very strong waves or movement of the atmospheric air. This effect is called the, 'Blast Effect'. It acts in the same way as an earthquake. The blast effect damages the lungs and eardrums if one stands in the direct line of the blast. The glass window panes are broken and glass splinters and other debris from the damaged houses fly in all directions. There have been more casualties caused by the flying debris, than by the direct hit of the high explosive bomb. Sometimes the bomb explodes after it has gone a little into the surface of the earth, in such a case, instead of a blast, the whole earth in the vicinity starts shaking. This is called the, 'Earth Shock Effect' and is responsible for damaging underground pipes, cables, sewage and other underground essential services. It also damages the foundations of the houses. Occasionally the bomb may fail to explode and would pose a problem, such a bomb will cause great fear in the minds of the people. Since the bomb may be lying buried or hidden and may be fitted with a short delay time or anti-disturbance type of fuse, it becomes very difficult to carry out the reconnaissance. Sometimes the bomb explodes below the ground leaving a hollow cavity known as comouflet which may be dangerously close to the surface of the ground and a person walking over it may collapse in it. The fallen person may suffocate by the poisonous fumes present after the explosion. The absence of explosion are positive signs of unexploded bomb, one may see part of the bomb or parachute lying nearby, please keep away from such objects. There are trained personnel like the Bomb Disposal Unit, who will arrange to dispose of these bomb.

Protection against High Explosive Bomb Attacks :

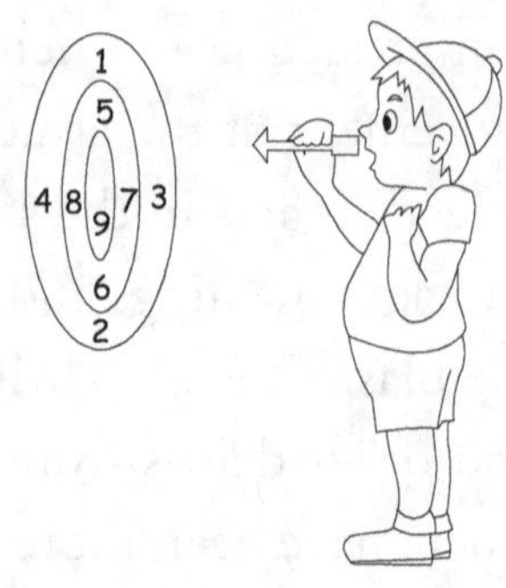

Warning of air raid will enable everyone to be prepared and take shelter. Due to the detection of the enemy aircraft by the radar, before it hit the actual targets, it gives enough time for the control room to sound a warning siren.

❁ On hearing the warning or the sound of the enemy bombers, do not run for cover if there is no time. Lie flat on the ground with face downward, keep chest slightly above the ground and rest on the elbows. Plug the ears with cotton and if cotton is not available, plug them with the corners of your kerchief. Never look up during an air raid.

❁ It is better to roll in a gutter or make a fold of your body on the ground, since the splinters and debris of the bomb fly in any direction either outward or upward.

❁ Never lean directly against the walls.

❁ Avoid being in the direct line of the door or windows.

❁ While travelling in a train, turn off the lights and crawl under the seats, do not look out of the windows.

❁ While travelling in a bus or a car, stop the vehicle and go out in the open.

❁ Prepare a refuge room in your own house, a room preferably on the ground floor with an overhead roof of reinforced concrete and the sidewalls preferably doubled. Ensure that the room is not too near the fire risk or water tank area.

Make arrangements for sanitary facilities and provide adequate drinking water facility, foodstuff, first aid equipment, torch, battery operated radio, rescue equipment like, rope, crowbar, pick, shovel, etc.

Incendiary Bomb:

It is a small container containing an incendiary agent (chemicals capable of catching fire immediately) like, Phosphorous, Thermite, Magnesium, etc. With the help of a fuse and High Explosive attachment, an Incendiary Bomb starts burning when it reaches the target and throws the burning material over a large area. The size of Incendiary bomb varies according to the requirement. Bomber planes carry these bombs and drop them from the air in racks, which open out before reaching the target. The bomb looks very violent and the damage created by the bomb cannot be extinguished by water and sand.

Protection against Incendiary Bomb attacks :

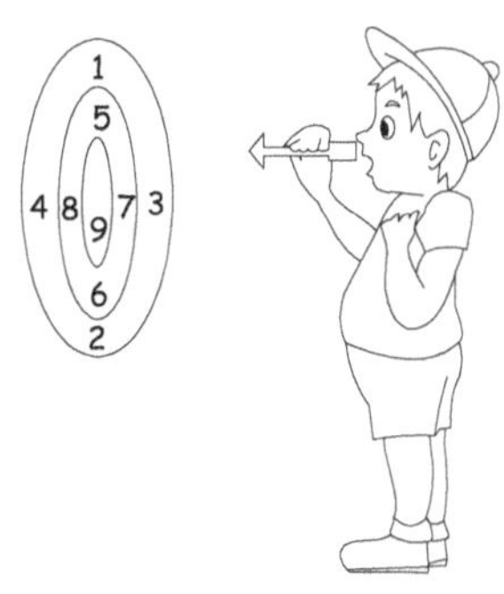

❊   Remove all inflammable material like old clothes, papers and rubbish from the roof of all the buildings.

❊   Keep all inflammable stores, which are essentially required, the rest to be dispersed as early as possible. This should also be done with all the stores in factories and industries.

❊   Use non-inflammable material as fire resistant on curtains, so that the material will not catch fire easily. A solution of one-gallon water, nine ounces of borax and four ounce of boric acid is very useful for dipping the curtains and other material to make it fire proof. Cover the ceiling if it is made of combustible material like wood, with sand.

   Arrange for reserve of water and sand near the place where one is likely to be in such an event.

Chapter : 13

‖ Psychological Warfare ‖

Victories are won when the will to survive and to make sacrifices for survival is maintained. If the morale is to be maintained, the general public should be protected from physical and psychological impacts. The most harmful undermines of morale are panic, rumours, rowdy behaviour and enemy propaganda under psychological warfare. Psychological warfare are wars fought in fourth dimension, i.e. people's minds, they are aimed to destroy the unity of peace-loving people, by misinterpreting the economic, social and cultural contacts amongst them and to arouse suspicion in their midst, to arouse deep-seated racial prejudices and thus create trouble by causing a wide-spread confusion, born out of fighting, non-cooperation and unfounded conflicts.

Things to do :

❀ Never spread rumours, always try to listen from authentic source. Discourage people who are on propaganda campaign, instead advice them to help the general public.

❀ Carry out evacuation procedures, and try to help the general public by giving first aid, food, clothing, and morale boosting.

Pets and Disaster

When disaster strikes it is important to take care of your pets. Take it with you where ever you move, if you cannot, make sure your pet can get into a safe, secure room without windows, but with adequate air (like a big bathroom). Leave enough food for three days. Leaving enough water for your pet is very important. One pet can drink several gallons of water a day. Put water in containers that are not easily knocked over. Leave the tap dripping into a bathtub or sink (with the drain open!). Leave their favourite bed and toys. Don't confine dogs and cats in the same space. Put a notice on your front door saying where your pets are in the house and a phone number where you will be. Never, ever leave your pet animal tied up outside!

Birds should be moved in a secure travel cage or carrier. If the weather is cold, wrap a blanket over the carrier and warm up the car first. During warm weather, carry a plant mister to mist the birds' feathers from time to time. Do not put water in the carrier, instead put a piece of fruit or vegetables with high water content. Keep a photo of your bird for identification. Try to keep the carrier in quiet place, but DO NOT let your pet out, as they may fly away in the confusion.

Lizards and other reptiles should be treated like birds. Snakes should be put in a pillowcase when they are evacuated. You will need to put them in a more secure place when you reach the evacuation site. If your snake requires regular feeding, carry food with you. And take a water bowl large enough for soaking your snake as well as a heating pad. Take bedding materials, food bowls and water bottles.

Animal Care Plan :

❂ Plan how your pets will be cared for if you have to evacuate, so have some animal shelters identified.

❂ Establish relationships with other animal owners in your neighborhood so in case you are not home, someone will be able to help your animal.

❂ Pets and service animals may become confused, panicked, frightened or disoriented during and after a disaster.

❂ Keep them confined or securely leashed or harnessed. A leash (or harness)is an important item for managing a nervous or upset animal.

❂ Assemble a kit for your service animal that will last seven days. Place it in a pack that your animal can carry (if it is large enough to do so) in case you need to evacuate.

The kit should include :
❂ A bowl for water and food.
❂ A seven-day supply of food.
❂ A blanket for bedding.
❂ Plastic bags and paper towels for disposing of feaces.
❂ Neosporin ointment for minor

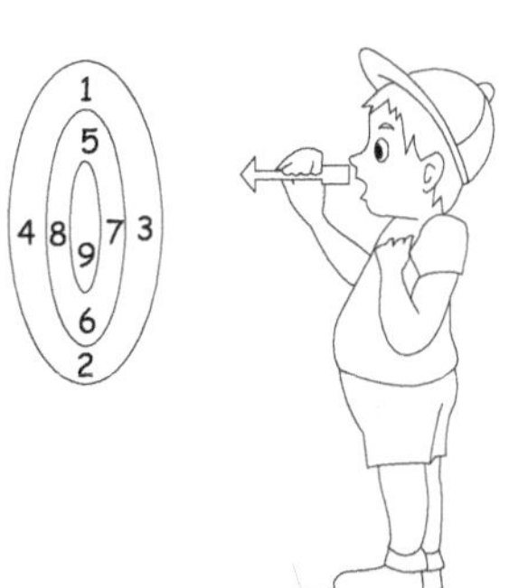

wounds. (Animals can easily get cut after an earthquake; ask your veterinarian if there is anything specific you should include for your animal).

* A favorite toy.
* An extra harness.

Chapter : 15

❚ Evacuation Techniques ❚

Evacuation techniques are the heart and soul of disaster management. It is the second stage in disaster management, also known as evacuation stage. Evacuation is done during and after the disaster period. No matter what age or caste, creed or sex does one belongs to, one has to know this skill of survival. Evacuating techniques comes in handy to evacuate the old, infirm, pregnant mother or lactating mother, the disabled, mentally or physically challenged, or the injured, depending upon the situation. Each life is precious, and it counts to make a city. We as human beings are joined in families, the families are joined in kinship groups, the kinship groups in clans, the clans in tribes, the tribes in nations, and that sense of hierarchy, of a pyramid in which layer upon layer is imposed. Hence life is precious, do take care.

Here are few of the techniques which could be handy, never go according to the set rules as mentiond below, but go according to what your heart and mind says, since the time and situation always keeps on changing and one has to accounts for his/her action, in the eyes of the higher SELF.

Precaution to be taken in time disaster :
- Remain cool and calm, even if you are trapped.
- In case of bombing or earthquake, try to take cover by getting under the table, chair or bed, see that you don't get crushed.

❀ It is better to be near the wall than in the center of the room.

❀ If caught within a house, which is on fire, try to escape through the windows by using ropes or bed sheet curtains, etc. to come down, after tying one end to a secure point. Incase there is no escape, try to call out for help by shouting, flag signalling, or through some source which could be handy, but never get panicky.

❀ Do not enter a damaged building, even if the situation appears to be most urgent. The time spent on such a survey is not a waste; one can't help anybody, if one himself/herself is injured.

❀ Wear a helmet or strong hat, or pagri, etc. for safety, since any loose element may come crashing on you.

❀ Always work in pairs, if entering a very narrow space, tie a chord around the waist and the other end to the partner, who is behind at a secure distance.

❀ Go on calling for casualty when searching. Listen to all types of sounds, this will facilitate location of casualties. Don't shout or scream unnecessary.

❀ Treat all naked electric wires as live.

❀ Walk or crawl close to the walls on a damaged staircase of upper floors. Keep off the debris.

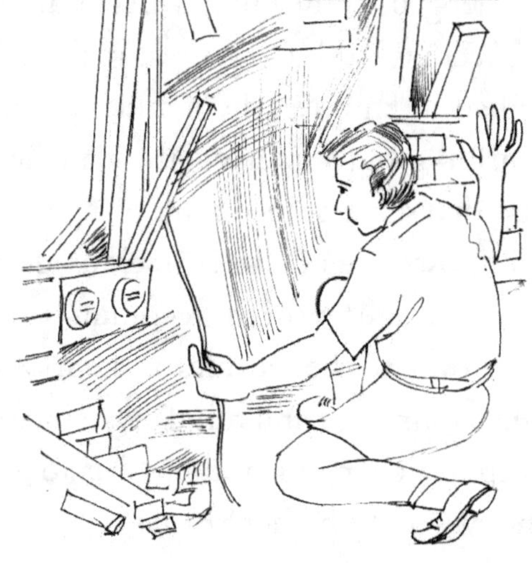

❀ In case the building is on fire, start the search for the trapped one from the top, since fire always moves upward. Search swiftly, but thoroughly.

❀ Do not forget to search under table, chairs, and bed or inside the cupboards, etc.

❁ Don't light a match or strike a lighter, in case the gas pipeline may have been damaged.

❁ Do not touch damaged walls or blocked doors, or disturb broken glass or door panes, since it could add to more casualties.

❁ Do not move carelessly and indiscriminately over the debris, do not pull timber. Look out for projecting nails and spikes, etc. If the debris

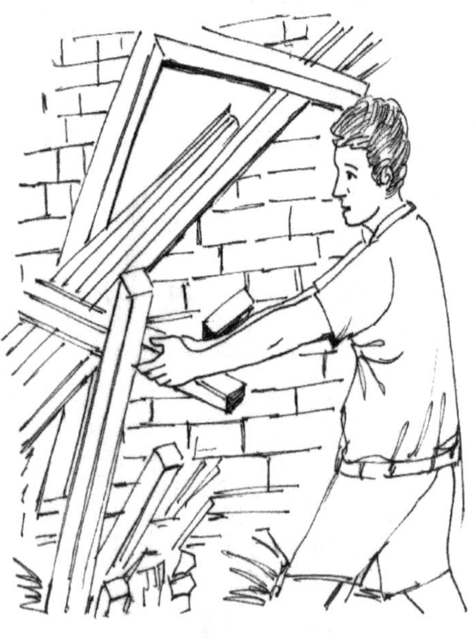

has to be removed to reach the casualty, then do it very carefully.

❁ If possible try to use ladders to rescue casualty from upper stories. Hold on to the rungs and not to the side of the ladder, Stand on the center of the rung and start climbing up, while climbing look up and not down.

Rescue Operations:

While rescuing a person from a disaster zone, one may be alone or accompanied by another partner. The following methods and techniques if followed can save the life of the victim without endangering oneself.

a) Human Crutch :

If the casualty can help himself, i.e. he is lightly hurt, then stand at his injured side, place the casualty's arm around the shoulder, grasping the wrist with your hand, pass the other hand around the casualty's waist gripping the clothing at the hip. Now assist him out of the dangerous site thus acting as a human crutch.

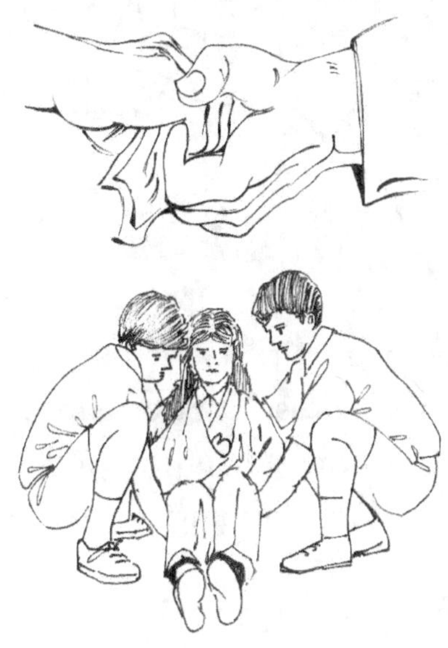

b)   Two handed seat method :

To carry an unconscious casualty with a partner to assist, face one another on either side of the casualty, pass each of your arms, which is nearest to the casualty's back, just below the shoulder, and if possible grip his clothing. Raise the casualty's back and each of you slip your other arm under the middle of the casualty's thigh clasping your hands with a hooking grip, pad your fingers with a handkerchief. Rise together and step off with short guided pace.

c)   Four-hand seat method :

If the casualty is conscious, stand facing each other, now each of you grip your own left wrist with your right hand. Now put your hand and your

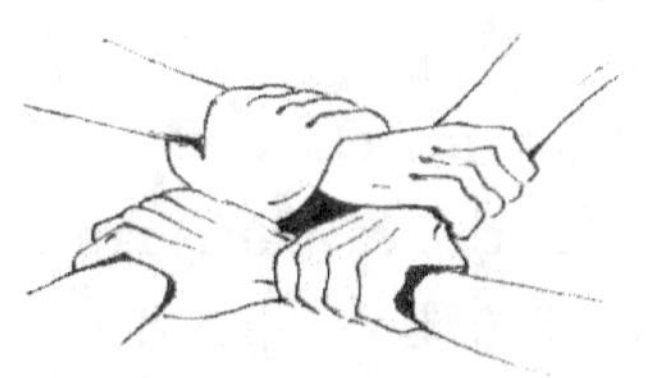

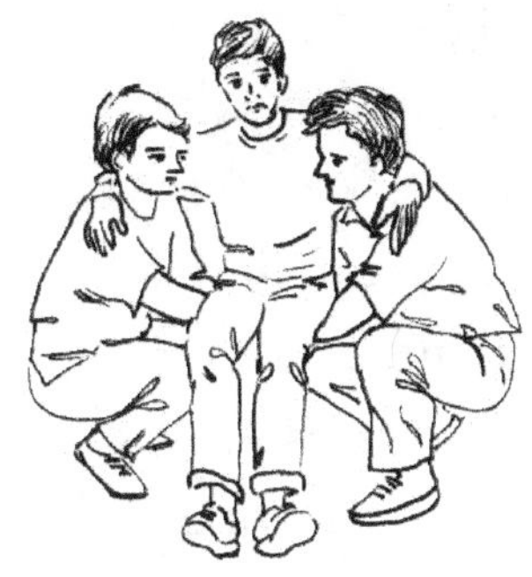 partner's hand together and each of you with your free left hand grasp the right wrist of each other. This will make a four-hand seat, place the casualty in the center and both his legs are in front of your respective hands and tell him to place his hands on your respective shoulders. Rise together and step with short guided pace. This method is excellent for a heavy individual.

d) Fore and Aft Method :

Place the casualty on his back, one of you raise the casualty shoulder and pass your hands under the arms from behind clasping him in front of the chest. The other partner takes one leg under each arm respectively and the casualty is carried feet first. If a leg is broken, both legs should be tied together or put in splints, and carried under one arm, instead of two arms.

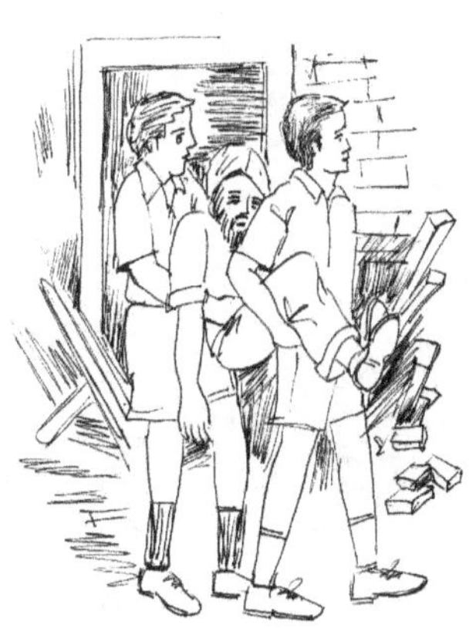

e) Fireman's lift (Method I) :

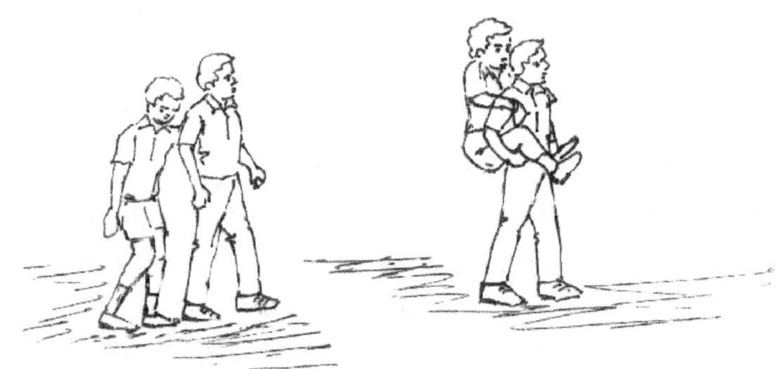

This technique can be used only by strong and well-balanced youth to help out the old, infirm and mentally challenged people. Stand in front of the casualty, by facing your back to him, then hold his both hands on top of your shoulder, then support his body by bending slightly in front, then lift his leg and bend it around your waist respectively. Place both your hands under his leg and near your waist and with body slightly bend start moving with a steady gait, towards a protective zone.

f)   Fireman's lift (Method II) :

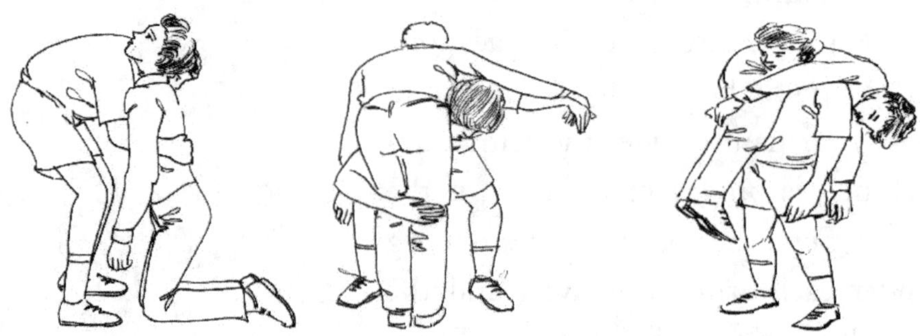

This method is used to move a conscious or unconscious child or a lightweight adult when you need to keep hands free. Help the casualty to stand up, if he is unconscious or unable to stand, turn him face down and stand at his head. Place the arms under his armpits and raise him on to his knees and then the feet. Grasp his right wrist with left hand, and bend down with your head under his extended right arm so that your shoulder is in level with his lower abdomen. Allow him to fall gently across your shoulders, place your right arm between or around his legs. Taking the weight on your right shoulder, stand up and gently pull him across both shoulders. Transfer his right wrist to your right hand, leaving your left hand free.

g) Fireman's crawl :

If the casualty is unconscious or too heavy or in a room full of smoke, turn him on his back and tie his wrist with a handkerchief, kneel astride facing him and place your head through the loop formed by his arms.

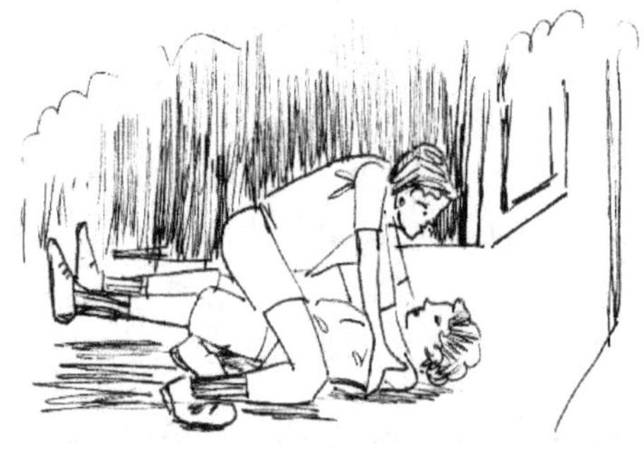

Crawl on your hands and knees and drag the casualty with you. While evacuating the casualty, try to tie a wet cloth over your mouth and nostril region, since the dampness may try to filter some of the toxic air. Remember air is heavier than gas, and gas always float above 18 inches from the floor.

h) Opening the door of a room on fire :

Fire produces a large amount of smoke, and the door of a room on fire should be opened with care as hot gases and smoke are bound to rush out. Crouch as low as possible and keep one foot away from the opening edge. Seek protection by the door itself and shut it again if necessary. If the door is not checked, the increased pressure in the room may cause it to burst open. You may tie a wet handkerchief on your mouth, and this will give protection against smoke.

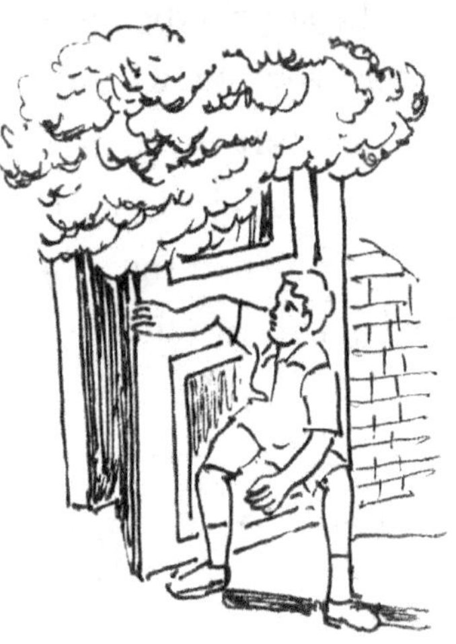

i)   **Chair Knot method :**

For rescuing people from heights, take a strong and long rope, grasp the rope in the center, with the left hand palm downwards, about a yard from the left hand, take the rope in the right hand palm upwards, turn the left hand palm upwards forming a loop (anticlockwise), turn the right hand palm down forming a loop. Pass the standing part through the loop of the opposite hand, by pulling them through, thus forming two loops with a knot in the center. Adjust the loop and make half hitch or a thumb knot on each loop. (Try to learn this knot from your Scout/Guide teacher). Place the casualty into the slings, the larger sling under the knees and the smaller sling under the armpits. Lower the casualty gently by moving the rope slowly, till he reaches down.

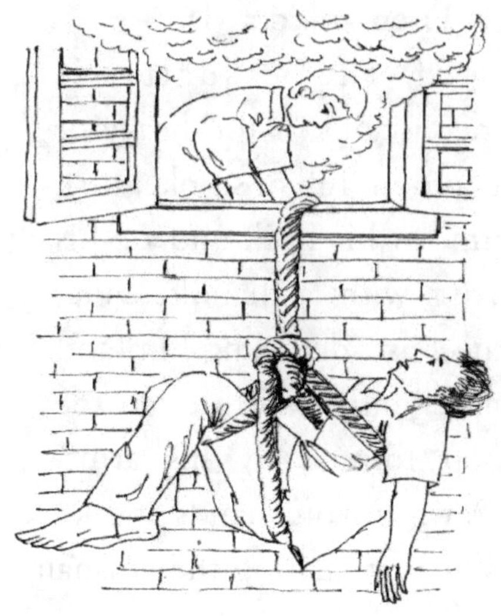

j)   **Charpoy (bed) as stretcher method two-point method :**

Secure the casualty to the charpoy, and secure four guide ropes to the four corners of the charpoy. Two guide ropes will be used for lowering the

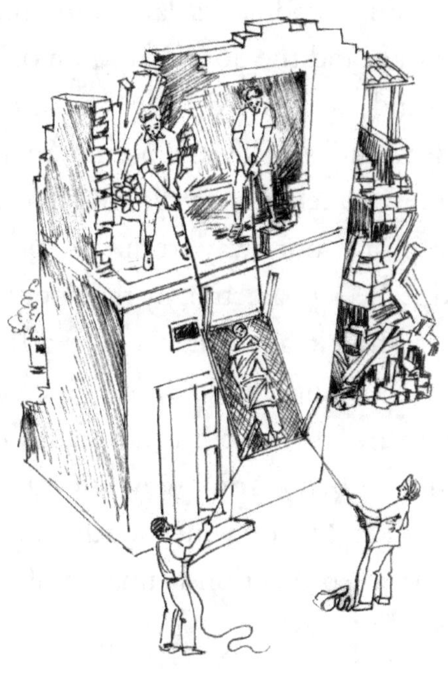

charpoy from an opening, whereas the other two guide ropes will be controlled by people standing down to receive the casualty.

k)   Charpoy (bed) as stretcher method four-point method :

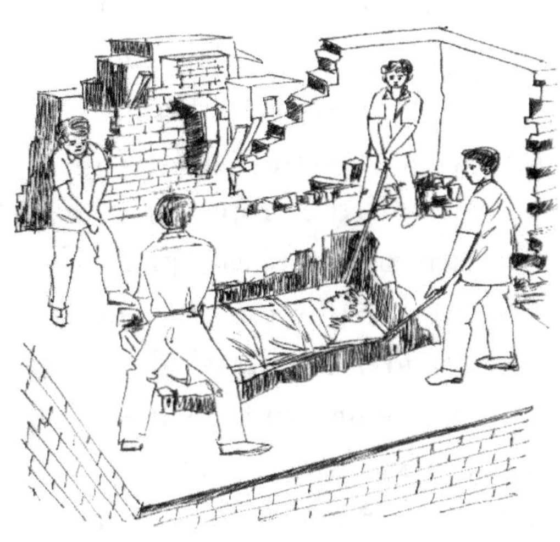

Secure the casualty to the charpoy, and secure four guide ropes to the four corners of the charpoy. Four people will lower the charpoy through the opening by loosening the rope simultaneously in well-guided synchronized actions. Whereas two more people who are standing down will receive the casualty and take the casualty to a more protective zone.

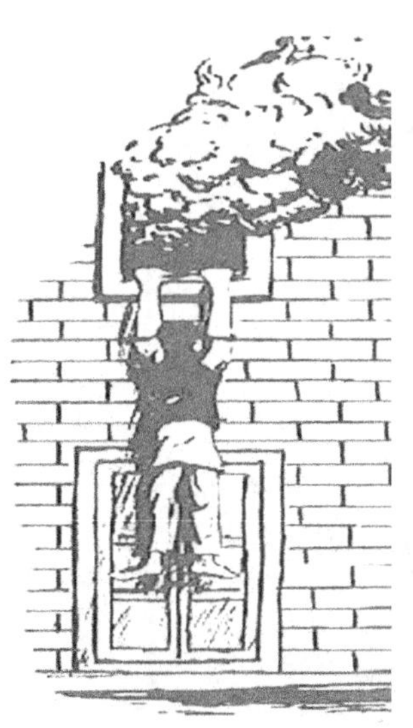

l) Escaping from first floor :

If you have to escape from a room on the first storey, sit on the window sill with your legs outside, turn over, slide down till you have a finger grip on the edge of the window sill and then let go. Do not jump, an adult can easily cut his fall by about seven feet (since his personal height is six feet and when the hand is stretched one gets another one to one and a half feet, the total becomes seven feet), he has to just lower his body to another four feet depending on the height of the flooring.

m) Escaping from second or third floor :

If you have to escape from a room on the second or third floor, tie some ropes or bed sheets, or curtains, etc. together and secure one end of the rope or the improvised rope to a heavy piece of furniture or a bathroom pipe, drop the other end out of the window or any other opening and slowly slide yourself down. Even if you are not able to reach the ground this way, you will reduce the drop by a great length and reach the ground with less chances of hurting yourself.

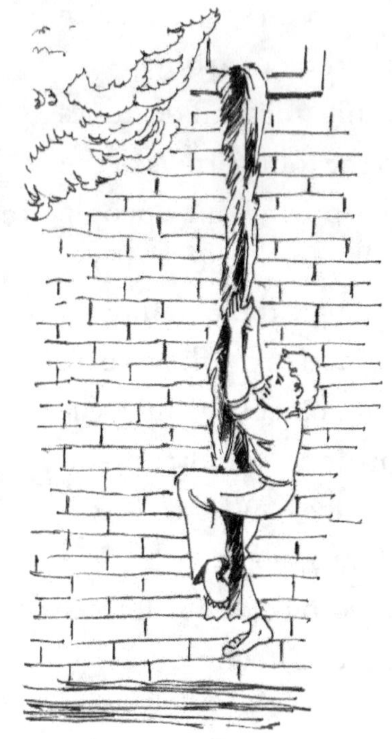

n) Chair method :

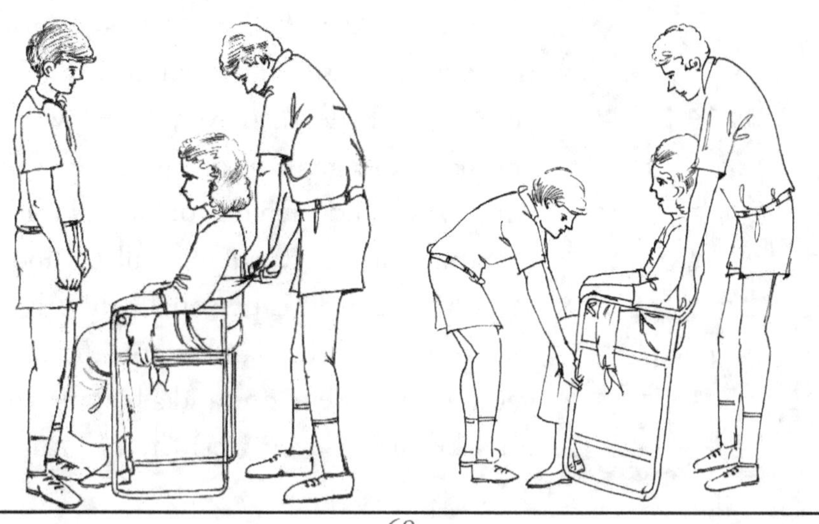

When a conscious casualty with no serious injuries is to be moved up or down stairs or along the passageways, the casualty can be seated on an ordinary chair and carried by two people. However, the passages must be cleared of any obstruction or dangers such as loose matting, etc. Test the chair to ensure it is strong, then place the casualty and secure it with 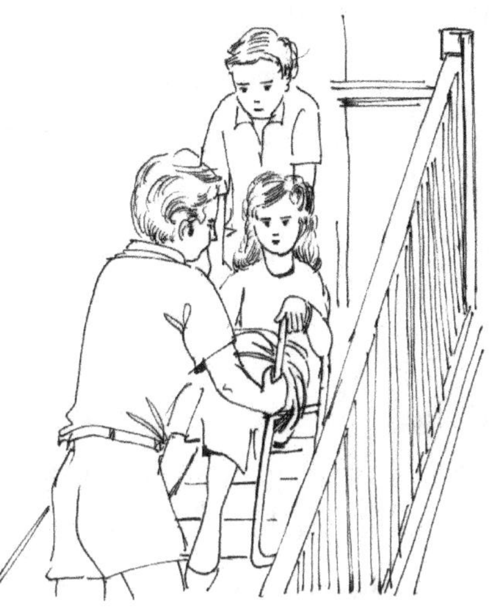 broad bandages. The person behind the chair should support the back of the chair and the casualty, the other should hold the chair by the front legs. Slowly tilt the chair backwards to seat the casualty, secure, and then lift together. With the casualty facing forwards, move slowly along the passage or stairs.

o)   **Blanket as stretcher :**

Roll the blanket or rug lengthwise for half its width, place the

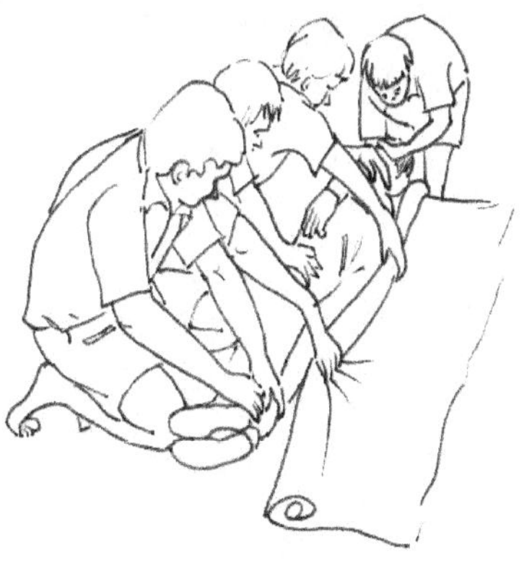 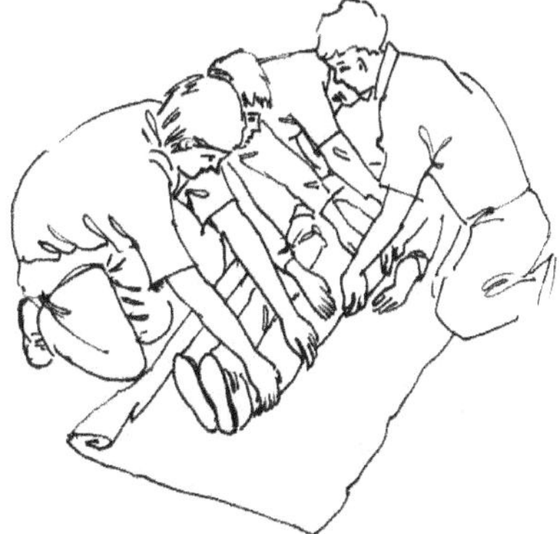

roll in line with the injured side of the casualty (or most severely injured side if both sides are injured). All four bearers should kneel at the side of the casualty, opposite to the blanket and turn the casualty slowly and gently on to the side towards them. Move the rolled portion of the blanket against the back. Gently turn the casualty on to the back over the roll 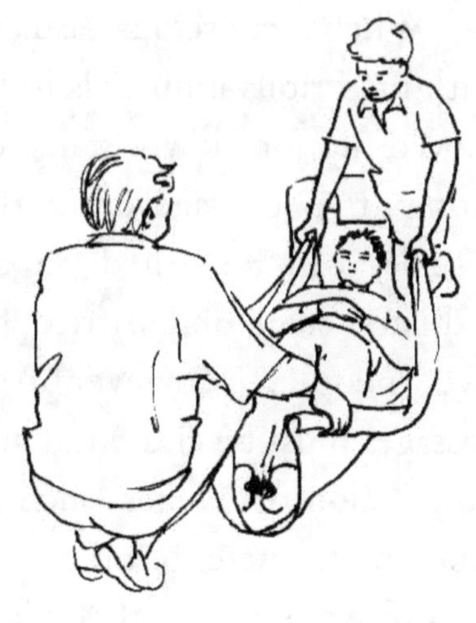 of blanket and turn the casualty far enough to the other side to allow the blanket to be unrolled. Now slowly lift the casualty and proceed to a safe zone.

p)   Improvised Stretchers :

An improvised stretcher can be made by the following procedure, tie broad-fold bandages at intervals around two strong

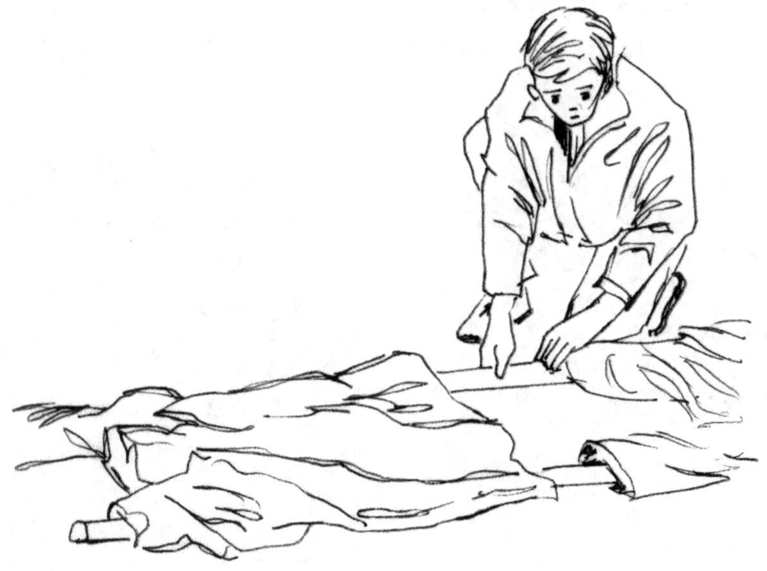

poles. Spread out a rug, piece of sack, tarapaulin or a strong blanket and roll up two strong poles at the sides. Use a worn out jacket's sleeves inside out, pass the two strong poles through the sleeves and button up the coats. The poles may be kept apart by strips of wood tied to the poles at each end of the stretcher.

Chapter : 16

‖ First Aid ‖

First aid is the third stage of disaster management or rehabilitation stage. After the disaster, one should be able to treat the sick and injured. During disaster thousands of people may be injured, but if you escape injury you can save the lives of others by giving first aid, before a qualified doctor arrives. Most of the injuries will be of a peculiar type of nature like, people getting cut from flying glass, some may receive burns injury, many cases of fracture of bones, many cases of bleeding or haemorrhage, many will have wounds and multiple injuries, some may have suffocation or unconsciousness. But remember: SHOCK WILL BE PRESENT IN ALMOST EVERY CASE.

Aim of giving First Aid :
- To preserve life.
- To prevent the casualty's condition worsening.
- To promote recovery and save a life.

Precaution to be taken before giving first add :
- Assess the situation without endangering one's own life.
- Identify the condition from which the casualty is undergoing.

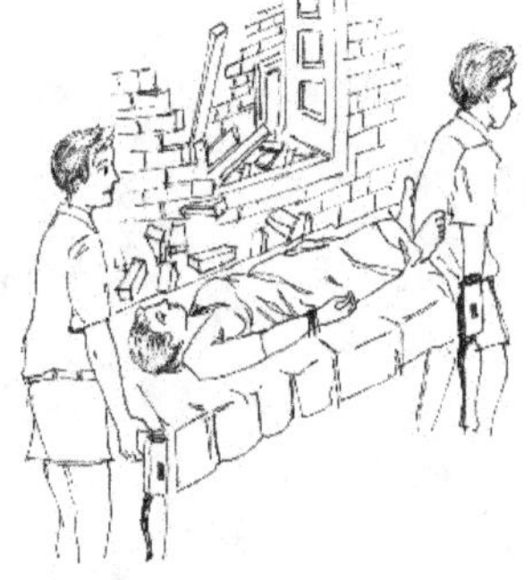

❀ If possible give immediate appropriate and adequate treatment. Always bear in mind that the casualty may have m o r e than one injury and that some casualties will require more urgent attention than others.

❀ Move the casualty out of the damaged building or the danger zone area or to an area where after shock effect is bare minimum, and there is no possibility of further collapse or any chance of fire to spread.

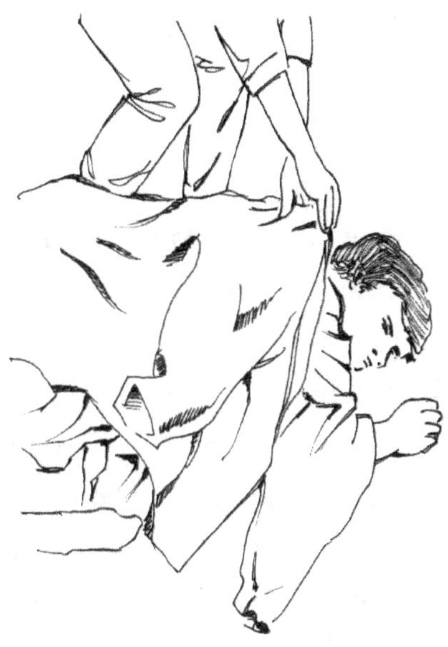

❀ Keep the casualty warm by using blankets or other cover, not for burnt casualties.

❀ If a casualty asks for a drink, give plain water, tea or coffee, unless there is a wound in the abdomen or any other danger for the food or liquid intake. Use your own discretion and see what is best at that situation.

❀ Be cheerful and keep the injured cheerful.

❀ Treat the injured as per required.

First Aid :

a) SHOCK :

Signs :

Faintness, paleness, weak pulse, weak breathing, perspiration especially on forehead region and cold extremities.

Treatment:

Stop the bleeding if present by applying ice or pressure techniques. Lay the casualty on the back, legs raised, loosen clothing, cover with blanket or coat, etc. Soothe him/her by reassuring words in a confident way. Support injured part, if any. DON'T GIVE ANY ALCOHOLIC DRINK.

b) WOUNDS :

Signs :

A wound is any cut which bleeds. It may be big or small, shallow or deep.

Treatment :

Cover it with clean dressing. Apply ice to stop bleeding, if ice is not available, then   keep the wound under a cold running water. If sterilized guaze is not available, fresh washed handkerchiefs, wels, sheets and sanitary pads, etc. will serve as dressing. Bandage the dressing on the wound very firmly to stop bleeding; eventies and scarves may be used as bandages. Do not put antiseptics like Iodine on a wound, and in case the bleeding does not stop, apply direct pressure.

C) BURNS :

Do's :

Pour water and try to bring the temperature of the burning limbs to as low as possible, give plenty of fluids. Immobilise the limb

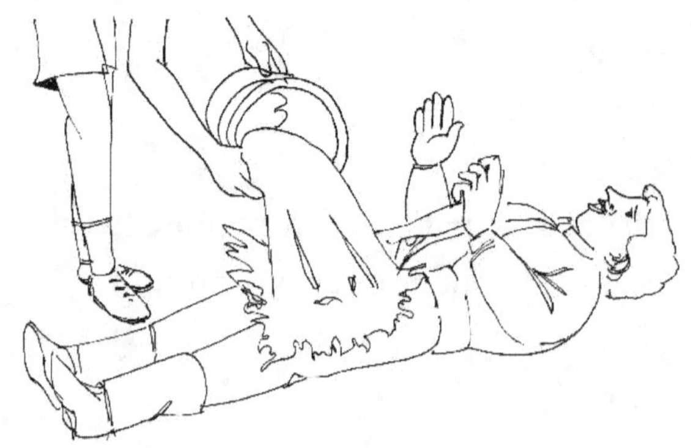

or the damage area with a well-padded splint. Raise the limb to diminish oozing of plasma. Cover the casualty with light clothing without making him/her sweat.

Don'ts :

Don't allow the casualty whose clothes are on fire to remain standing. If the casualty starts running, trip him/her at once, before more damage is done. Don't roll him on the floor, or throw any thick towel or blanket on him, instead douse the flame with cold water. Do not open the blisters; do not attempt to clean the burnt area. Do not apply any greasy ointments or powder, since you will be giving fuel to the burnt area to burn more.

d) FRACTURES :

Signs :

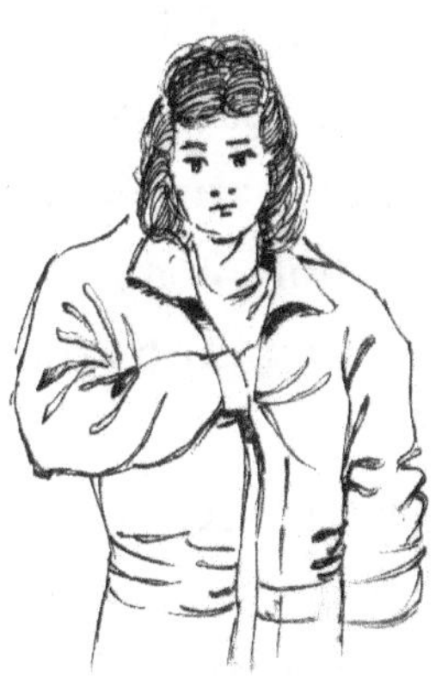

Pain and tenderness of the fractured limb, loss of power in the fractured limb, deformity of the limb, there may be slight swelling, or shortening of the limb. Abnormal mobility.

Treatment :

Do not move the casualty without treating the fracture, put splints or give support to the fractured limb, since this will stop further damage. Folded bundle of newspaper, umbrella or stick will serve the purpose. Make the patient comfortable, handle and move the patient as little as possible. Guard against shock and stop bleeding if any. If there is bleeding then cover the wound with a dressing. A broken arm should be suspended from neck by a sling. Broken leg should be tied to the other leg. Do not remove any clothing, but cut it away incase if it hampers the movement. **Do not attempt to set the bone.**

e) SUFFOCATION :

Signs :

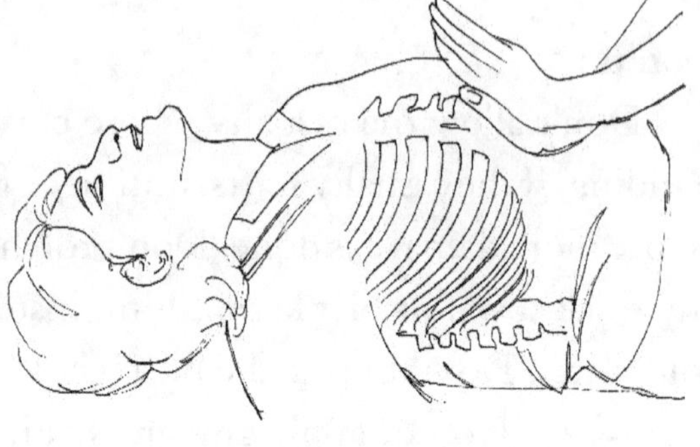

Gasping for breath, restlessness, face livid, lips and fingernails are blue, eyes blood shot red and staring, veins in the neck standing out.

Treatment :

Remove the cause or source of the danger or the casualty from the source of danger. Clear the air passage, i.e. mouth, nose and throat. Loosen clothing around chest, waist and neck. Keep the casualty warm, cover with blankets if necessary. Ensure free circulation of air. If required give artificial respiration, if possible give thumping on the chest it may revive the casualty.

f) ARTIFICIAL RESPIRATION :

Begin the procedure immediately, since every second counts, place the patient face downwards, with forehead resting on hands

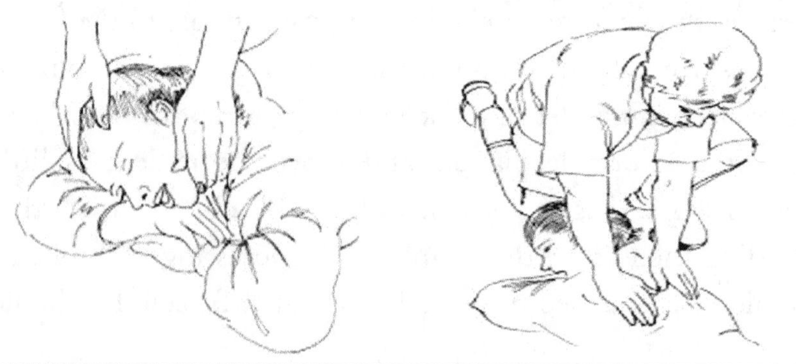

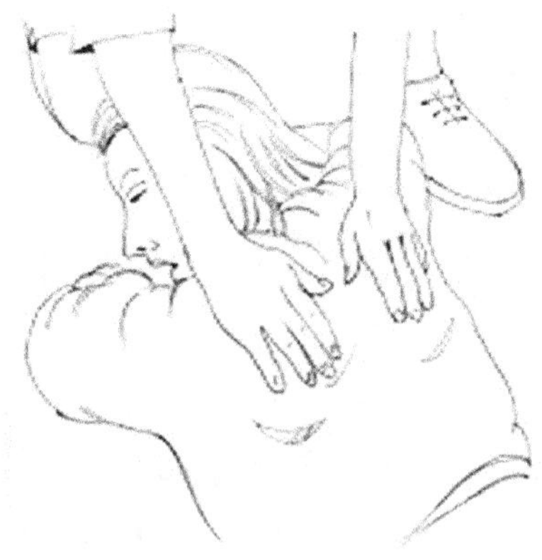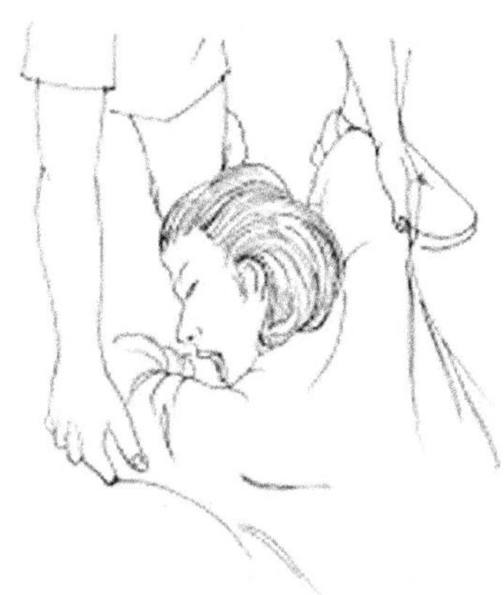

placed one top of the other. The
mouth and nose must be kept free of the ground. Bring the
patient's tongue forward by firmly slapping in between the
shoulder blade, with the base of your palm, or by applying pressure
in between the shoulder blade. Kneel on one knee and a little in
front of the patient's head, while the other knee near the patient
elbow. Your midline should be in alignment with the patients
spinal chord. Now hold the patients elbow and rock slightly
forward on the outstretched arms until they are vertical. The
pressure should be light, without force (about 10 kgs.), this will
induce respiration.

g) Mouth-to-Mouth Ventilation :

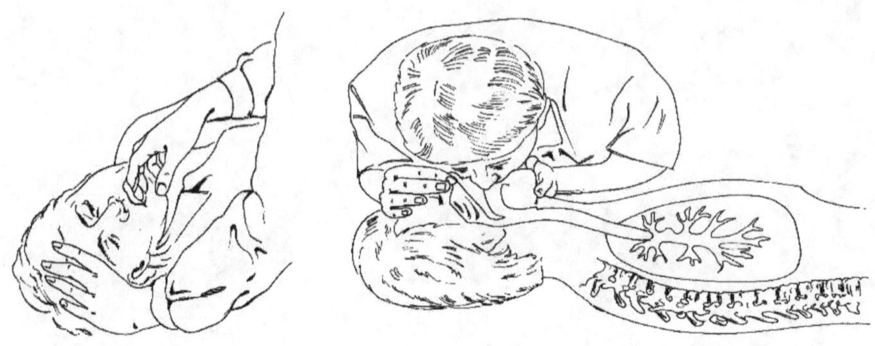

This is the most preferred method of artificial ventilation in all cases. If the mouth cannot be used, satisfactorly ventilation can be achieved through the nose (mouth-to-nose). Remove any obstructions over the face or constrictions around the neck. Open the airway and remove any debris seen in the mouth or throat. Open your mouth wide, take a deep breath, pinch the casualty's nostrils together with your fingers and seal your lips around his mouth. Blow into the casualty's lungs, looking along his chest, until you can see his chest rise to maximum expansion (if the casualty's chest fails to rise, first assume his airway is not fully open, adjust the position of his head and jaw and try again). Remove your mouth well away from the casualty's and breathe out any excess air while watching his chest fall. Take a deep breath, repeat inflation. After two inflations, check the pulse to make sure the heart is beating. If the

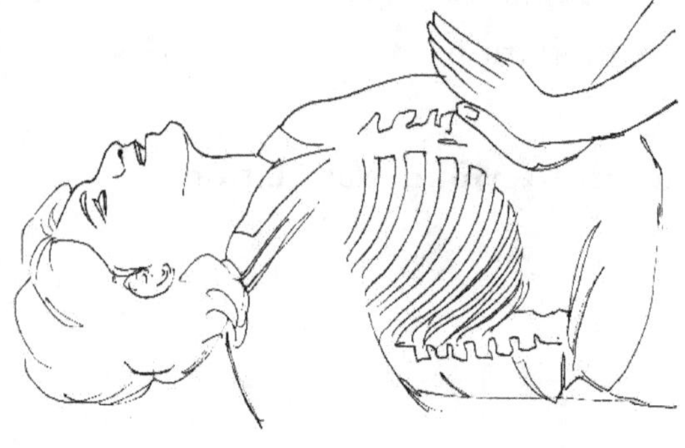

heart is beating and a pulse is felt, continue to give inflations at a rate 12 to 16 times per minute until natural breathing is restored. Don't be panicky, you may feel that you are filling the patient with your own carbon dioxide, but in reality the atmosphere contains 20% of Oxygen, out of which we inhale only 4% and the rest 16% of Oxygen is exhaled, and this exhaled Oxygen can revive the patient. If the heart is not beating you must perform external chest compression immediately.

Chapter : 17

▌▌ Benefits of Disaster Management ▌▌

Benefits of Disaster Management to students, parents, teachers and society at large :

- Children will learn how to take care of home, school as well as national property, e.g. they can check seepage, leakage, unsafe electric connections, etc. This will enable to utilize c o m m u n i t y resources in a fruitful manner.

- Students who become familiar with disaster management techniques, will themselves be add on hand, to ensure adequate facilities and relief.

- Students will plant trees and create shelterbelts for the school, which in turn is also an environment improvemental measure.

- They will understand the fragile balance of eco-system and environment, and tend to maintain it.

- Students will be in touch with local fire brigades, ambulance services and other emergency services and in the process improve the safety of school and their loved one.

- Students will become aware and feel the need for physical fitness; hence they will get involve in Physical Training and Games Period.

- They will learn skills like earthquake and fire drills, sounding alert, helping people in the face of danger, all with a smile. Hence panic and commotion will be under control, rescue operation and evacuation techniques can be applied during time of disaster.

- While working for relief operation, students will be exposed and interacting with people from various different sector of society like Law and Order, Judiciary, NGO's, Local Civil Defence, Hospitals, Local Fire Brigade, etc. This will bring out attitudinal change and act as a great motivator for the children.

- The exposure to practical and useful skills will give them a wide choice in their career hunt. Their productivity will enhance many-fold, besides practical skills will also enrich their Science and Social Studies subject.

- Preparation of projects and planning are essential steps in Disaster Management training, these skills will benefit the students in future. In adult life they will be able to give vital suggestions and build strong proposals to build better life for the citizen of this nation and develop strong human resources.

- A sense of belonging to the community and nation will develop the process of halting the brain drain situation that is taking rapidly over this country.

▌▌ **Bibliography** ▌▌

1. Civil Defence for Householders, by Government Of India, Directorate General of Civil Defence, 1950, Delhi.

2. First Aid Manual, by St. John Ambulance, St. Andrew's Ambulance association, and the British Red Cross Society, London, U.K.

3. Textbook of Disaster Management for Class IX, by Goyal Brothers Prakashan, 2005, New Delhi.

‖ About the Authors ‖

Dr. Fr. Francis Swamy s.j., born in 1955, a great educationist and involved most of the time for the betterment of the youth. He was the Principal of Holy Family High School, Andheri 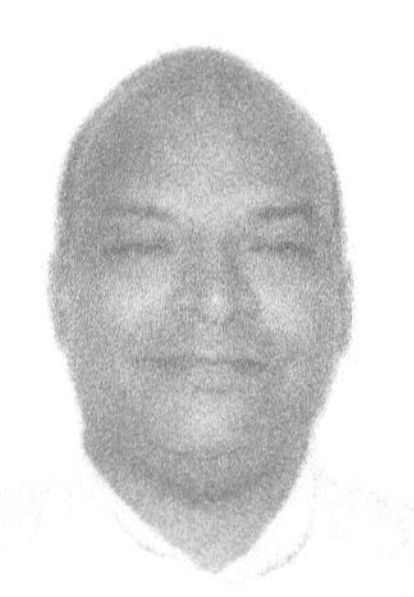(E), Mumbai for the last five years. Dr. Fr. Francis Swamy s.j. was the member of Maharashtra State Board of Higher and Secondary Education, Mumbai Division. Dr. Fr. Francis Swamy s.j. is continuously involved in betterment of the youth, and society at large, hence he is involved with various groups and still is the Member of the famous social service group called the, 'Agni Swyamsevaka Sangh'. He is the convenor of the 'Inter Religious Prayer Group', member of the social service group called the, 'Mohalla Committee' and the member of the, 'Saki Naka Citizen Quorum'. He is the trustee of, 'Ashankur Welfare Centre', Andheri (E), Sub-Convenor of K-East Ward, and Executive Officer by the Government of Maharashtra.

Being involved with the students and various youth groups, and simultaneously as a youth he had participated in many of the Social Service League programmes and being in the NCC has given him an extra edge to understand the demand of modern youth. The recent disaster has made him think of how to handle disaster and train the youth in the subject of Disaster Management for posterity.

E-mail   :   francisswamy@rediffmail.com

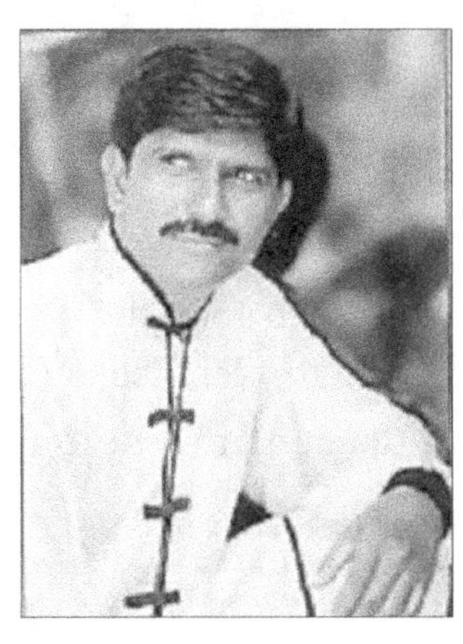

Mr. Christopher Fernandes, born in 1962 a trained martial art exponent in the field of 'Hua-Chuan Kung-Fu', trained by the late Lama Sevang Migyuar Nobu. Mr. Christopher Fernandes became the first Indian to be trained in Beijing, People's Republic of China. In 1988 he founded the Universal Martial Arts Research Centre, where an extensive research, data compiling was done in Indian Martial Arts. In 1993 he was the official observer for the Second World Wu-Shu Meet at Kuala Lumpur in Malayasia. From 1995 till 2003 he conducted martial arts tournaments in different streams (such as judo, karate, wu-shu, and tae kwon do) at the grass root level for school children under the auspices body of the Mumbai School Sports Association, which is the oldest sporting body in the world. He choreographs martial arts sequences for commercial ads, TV serials, films, and simultaneously coaches many of the film stars from Mumbai, in Chinese Martial Arts. During the last 25 years he has trained scores of students including security personnel, paramilitary forces, and civilians in armed & unarmed combat, and stress relieving techniques such as Tai Chi Chuan and Qi Gong. His earlier four books were great successes, both at home and abroad. They are as follows:

❀ "The Art of Kung Fu Wu Shu", published by Zorba Publishers, the second edition was published by English Edition and was titled "Chinese Martial Arts",

❀ "The Art of Stick Fighting", published by Zorba Publishers,

❀ "Tai Chi Chuan The Mantra for Health and Fitness", published

by Zorba Publishers,

 "The Art of Self Defence", published by English Edition, foreword by J.F.Ribeiro (Ex. Director General of Police).

He lives and teaches in Mumbai, India. He is currently working in Holy Family High School, Andheri (E), as a teacher for the last 17 years. Being involved in Scouting, Civil Defence and Martial Arts has given him an extra edge to understand the subject of Disaster Management better.

Voice mail   :   91-80825 55543

E-mail   :   chris@sevangee.com